OVER 50 COVID-19 BIOMARKERS EXACERBATED BY GLUCOSE, AND POTENTIALLY IMPROVED BY CANNABINOIDS, CURCUMIN, VITAMIN D, AND GABA: RESULTS OF AN ONGOING DATABASE SEARCH

8/01/2022

Russell Redden

The Rogue Researcher

ISBN: 9798847240802

OVER 50 COVID-19 BIOMARKERS EXACERBATED BY GLUCOSE, AND POTENTIALLY IMPROVED BY CANNABINOIDS, CURCUMIN, VITAMIN D, AND GABA: RESULTS OF AN ONGOING DATABASE SEARCH
8/01/2022

Russell Redden
The Rogue Researcher
Mesa, Colorado
Cannabinoid research

Abstract:
Based on recent reports that the supplements CBD, Curcumin, Vitamin D, and GABA could be potential treatments for COVID-19, and reports of high glucose, and obesity being a major factor in fatalities, a data base search of over 600 genes, enzymes, proteins, and other substances affected by COVID-19 was begun, first on those that are major triggers of SARS-COV-2, or implicated in "long" or "severe" COVID. Search terms, including but not limited to: "CBD" "THC" "cannabis" "curcumin," "vitamin-d" "GABA (γ-Aminobutyric Acid)" and "glucose," are currently being conducted in the PUBMED database. This document presents the initial results.

Results:
So far, almost universally, over 50 biomarkers aggregated by COVID-19 are also made worse by high glucose, and potentially improved by all four of these supplements, according to, but not limited to, in vivo, and in Vitro studies. Considering clinical trials have been conduced on some drugs that have had some positive outcomes on only a less than a dozen of these biomarkers, the 54 presented in this document should be more than enough evidence to warrant clinical trials on a combined treatment strategy using these supplements. This evidence is not limited to lab tests, but also clinical trials unrelated to COVID-19 [1] [2] [3].

These supplements either independently, or together, should perform all of the things necessary in the treatment of COVID-19 [4]: limiting viral entry; reducing the cytokine storm; reducing blood coagulation and vascular damage; and preventing lung injury. And since the coronavirus uses sugar to replicate [5], which raises cytokine levels [6], and the COVID-19

---

1 Wessam Mustafa, Nadia Elgendy, Samer Salama, Mohamed Jawad, Khaled Eltoukhy, "The Effect of Cannabis on the Clinical and Cytokine Profiles in Patients with Multiple Sclerosis", Multiple Sclerosis International, vol. 2021, Article ID 6611897, 10 pages, 2021. https://doi.org/10.1155/2021/6611897

2 Gupta SC, Patchva S, Aggarwal BB. Therapeutic roles of curcumin: lessons learned from clinical trials. AAPS J. 2013 Jan;15(1):195-218. doi: 10.1208/s12248-012-9432-8. Epub 2012 Nov 10. PMID: 23143785; PMCID: PMC3535097.

3 Yusupov E, Li-Ng M, Pollack S, Yeh JK, Mikhail M, Aloia JF. Vitamin d and serum cytokines in a randomized clinical trial. Int J Endocrinol. 2010;2010:305054. doi: 10.1155/2010/305054. Epub 2010 Aug 12. PMID: 20871847; PMCID: PMC2943086.

4 Aigner, Ludwig et al. "The Leukotriene Receptor Antagonist Montelukast as a Potential COVID-19 Therapeutic." Frontiers in molecular biosciences vol. 7 610132. 17 Dec. 2020, doi:10.3389/fmolb.2020.610132

5 Nguyen, L., McCord, K.A., Bui, D.T. et al. Sialic acid-containing glycolipids mediate binding and viral entry of SARS-CoV-2. Nat Chem Biol 18, 81–90 (2022). https://doi.org/10.1038/s41589-021-00924-1

6 Esposito K, Nappo F, Marfella R, Giugliano G, Giugliano F, Ciotola M, Quagliaro L, Ceriello A, Giugliano D. Inflammatory cytokine concentrations are acutely increased by hyperglycemia in humans: role of oxidative stress. Circulation. 2002 Oct 15;106(16):2067-72. doi: 10.1161/01.cir.0000034509.14906.ae. PMID: 12379575.

virus itself elevates blood sugar, even in those who do not have diabetes [7], a diet low in sugars and reduced carbs should also be simultaneously implemented.

Completion: This database search is ongoing, until all of these substances can be cross-referenced and evaluated in the database of the National Library of Medicine, and other medical journals, using this search criteria.

Introduction

COVID-19 affects more than 600 genes, releasing cytokines, enzymes, proteins, and other substances that can be harmful in excess, or cause problems if lowered in production. According the data in this document, over 50 of these biomarkers could be improved (reduced or enhanced) by four inexpensive, easily obtainable supplements. Conversely, glucose, sugar intake, and obesity almost universally makes these biomarkers worse. The endocrine society has recommended to limit sugar intake during COVID-19 infection [8] This is because high glucose is related to the severity of COVID-19, proven by numerous studies cited in this document. Despite this fact, this important diet recommendation is missing from COVID-19 hospital protocols [9] written by the National Institutes of Health (NIH,) and dispensed through the Food and Drug Administration (FDA,) and the Center for Disease Control (CDC.) In the search for "COVID-19 guidance," the term "sugar" brought up no results as of 07/29/22. The CDC has warned in statements that diabetes and obesity are risk factors, but if hospital protocols do not limit sugar intake, or if people suffering from COVID-19 at home do not know this important fact, failure to include this information might have contributed to COVID-19 fatalities.

Due to the fact glucose almost universally makes these biomarkers worse, failure to limit sugar intake in clinical trials could potentially skew results of any studies conducted either individually, or collectively, on these supplements. For this reason, clinical trials should combine our present knowledge about glucose when testing the effects of either supplements or medications in clinical trials.

The analysis so far

Viral entry and propagation

1. ACE2 (angiotensin-converting enzyme 2)
"The angiotensin converting enzyme-2 (ACE-2) has been identified as the receptor for the SARS-CoV-2 viral entry. As such, it is now receiving renewed attention as a potential target for anti-viral therapeutics. We review the physiological functions of ACE2 in the cardiovascular system and the lungs, and how the activation of ACE2/MAS/G protein coupled receptor

---

7 Carrasco-Sánchez FJ, López-Carmona MD, Martínez-Marcos FJ, Pérez-Belmonte LM, Hidalgo-Jiménez A, Buonaiuto V, Suárez Fernández C, Freire Castro SJ, Luordo D, Pesqueira Fontan PM, Blázquez Encinar JC, Magallanes Gamboa JO, de la Peña Fernández A, Torres Peña JD, Fernández Solà J, Napal Lecumberri JJ, Amorós Martínez F, Guisado Espartero ME, Jorge Ripper C, Gómez Méndez R, Vicente López N, Román Bernal B, Rojano Rivero MG, Ramos Rincón JM, Gómez Huelgas R; SEMI-COVID-19 Network. Admission hyperglycaemia as a predictor of mortality in patients hospitalized with COVID-19 regardless of diabetes status: data from the Spanish SEMI-COVID-19 Registry. Ann Med. 2021 Dec;53(1):103-116. doi: 10.1080/07853890.2020.1836566. PMID: 33063540; PMCID: PMC7651248.
8 Anuraag A Vazirani, COVID-19, an Incentive to Tackle Sugar in Hospitals and at Home, Journal of the Endocrine Society, Volume 5, Issue 6, June 2021, bvab037, https://doi.org/10.1210/jendso/bvab037
9 https://files.covid19treatmentguidelines.nih.gov/guidelines/covid19treatmentguidelines.pdf

contributes in reducing acute injury and inhibiting fibrogenesis of the lungs and protecting the cardiovascular system..” *(ACE2, Much More Than Just a Receptor for SARS-COV-2)*[10] *.”*

Covid-19 Binds to the ACE2 Receptor
Role of angiotensin-converting enzyme 2 (ACE2) in COVID-19 [11]

Sugar Helps the Coronavirus Bind to the Ace2 Receptor
Characterization of ACE and ACE2 Expression within Different Organs of the NOD Mouse [12]

Cannabinoid Likely Suppress ACE2 Replication in the Lungs.(Preprint)
Cannabidiol Inhibits SARS-CoV-2 Replication and Promotes the Host Innate Immune Response [13]

Curcumin Likely Suppresses Replication in ACE2 Receptors
Catechin and curcumin interact with S protein of SARS-CoV2 and ACE2 of human cell membrane: insights from computational studies [[14]]

Vitamin D Likely Suppresses Replication in ACE2 Receptors
A brief review of interplay between vitamin D and angiotensin-converting enzyme 2: Implications for a potential treatment for COVID-19[15]

Gaba Decreases ACE2 Expression
ACE2 modulates glucose homeostasis through GABA signaling during metabolic stress[16]

2. CD47

“CD47 (also known as the integrin-associated signal transducer) is a cell surface molecule in the immunoglobulin superfamily that has been reported to bind to several different proteins, including integrins (Brown & Frazier, 2001), thrombospondin-1 (Gao et al., 1996), and most importantly, signal regulatory protein α (SIRPα) (Tsai & Discher, 2008), which is a heavily glycosylated transmembrane protein with an immunoreceptor tyrosine-based inhibition motif (ITIM).”[17].”

Covid-19 infects via CD47
Targeting innate immunity by blocking CD14: Novel approach to control inflammation and organ dysfunction in COVID-19 illness[18]

CD47 causes insulin resistance

10 Samavati L, Uhal BD. ACE2, Much More Than Just a Receptor for SARS-COV-2. Front Cell Infect Microbiol. 2020 Jun 5;10:317. doi: 10.3389/fcimb.2020.00317. PMID: 32582574; PMCID: PMC7294848.

11 Ni, W., Yang, X., Yang, D. et al. Role of angiotensin-converting enzyme 2 (ACE2) in COVID-19. Crit Care 24, 422 (2020). https://doi.org/10.1186/s13054-020-03120-0

12 Roca-Ho H, Riera M, Palau V, Pascual J, Soler MJ. Characterization of ACE and ACE2 Expression within Different Organs of the NOD Mouse. Int J Mol Sci. 2017 Mar 5;18(3):563. doi: 10.3390/ijms18030563. PMID: 28273875; PMCID: PMC5372579.

13 Nguyen, Long Chi et al. “Cannabidiol Inhibits SARS-CoV-2 Replication and Promotes the Host Innate Immune Response.” bioRxiv : the preprint server for biology 2021.03.10.432967. 10 Mar. 2021, doi:10.1101/2021.03.10.432967. Preprint.

14 Jena, A.B., Kanungo, N., Nayak, V. et al. Catechin and curcumin interact with S protein of SARS-CoV2 and ACE2 of human cell membrane: insights from computational studies. Sci Rep 11, 2043 (2021). https://doi.org/10.1038/s41598-021-81462-7

15 Malek Mahdavi, Aida. “A brief review of interplay between vitamin D and angiotensin-converting enzyme 2: Implications for a potential treatment for COVID-19.” Reviews in medical virology vol. 30,5 (2020): e2119. doi:10.1002/rmv.2119

16 Ma X, Gao F, Chen Q, Xuan X, Wang Y, Deng H, Yang F, Yuan L. ACE2 modulates glucose homeostasis through GABA signaling during metabolic stress. J Endocrinol. 2020 Sep;246(3):223-236. doi: 10.1530/JOE-19-0471. PMID: 32698150.

17 Lisha Xiang, Gregg L. Semenza, in Advances in Cancer Research, 2019

18 Thomas R. Martin, Mark M. Wurfel, Ivan Zanoni, Richard Ulevitch, Targeting innate immunity by blocking CD14: Novel approach to control inflammation and organ dysfunction in COVID-19 illness, EbioMedicine, Volume 57, 2020, 102836, ISSN 2352-3964, https://doi.org/10.1016/j.ebiom.2020.102836.

Soluble CD14 and CD14 Variants, Other Inflammatory Markers, and Glucose Dysregulation in Older Adults: The Cardiovascular Health Study[19]

Cannabinoids reduce CD47

Δ9-tetrahydrocannabinol treatment during human monocyte differentiation reduces macrophage susceptibility to HIV-1 infection[20]

Curcumin reduces CD47

The Role Of Curcumn In Human Dendritic Cell Maturation And Function[21]

Vitamin D reduces CD47

Vitamin D₃ derivatives increase soluble CD14 release through ERK1/2 activation and decrease IL-8 production in intestinal epithelial cells[22]

Gaba: no data found

3. GABA (Gamma-aminobutyric acid). "Gaba is well known as a main inhibitory neurotransmitter in the central nervous system. Its physiological roles are related to the modulation of synaptic transmission, the promotion of neuronal development and relaxation, and the prevention of sleeplessness and depression. Besides, various pharmaceutical properties of Gaba on non-neuronal peripheral tissues and organs were also reported due to anti-hypertension, anti-diabetes, anti-cancer, antioxidant, anti-inflammation, anti-microbial, anti-allergy, hepato-protection, reno-protection, and intestinal protection. Therefore, Gaba may be considered as potential alternative therapeutics for prevention and treatment of various diseases. [23]."

Covid-19 reduces Gaba. This has been proposed as a major route of initial infection.
Disturbed lipid and amino acid metabolisms in COVID-19 patients[24]

High Glucose inhibits Gaba

Glucose inhibits GABA release by pancreatic beta-cells through an increase in GABA shunt activity[25]

Prolonged Cannabinoid Exposure increase GABA.

Prolonged cannabinoid exposure alters GABA(A) receptor mediated synaptic function in cultured hippocampal neurons[26]

19 Shitole SG, Biggs ML, Reiner AP, Mukamal KJ, Djoussé L, Ix JH, Barzilay JI, Tracy RP, Siscovick D, Kizer JR. Soluble CD14 and CD14 Variants, Other Inflammatory Markers, and Glucose Dysregulation in Older Adults: The Cardiovascular Health Study. Diabetes Care. 2019 Nov;42(11):2075-2082. doi: 10.2337/dc19-0723. Epub 2019 Aug 30. PMID: 31471378; PMCID: PMC6804612.

20 Williams, Julie C et al. "Δ(9)-Tetrahydrocannabinol treatment during human monocyte differentiation reduces macrophage susceptibility to HIV-1 infection." Journal of neuroimmune pharmacology : the official journal of the Society on NeuroImmune Pharmacology vol. 9,3 (2014): 369-79. doi:10.1007/s11481-014-9527-3

21 Shirley, Shawna A., "The Role Of Curcumin In Human Dendritic Cell Maturation And Function" (2008). Graduate Theses and Dissertations.
    https://digitalcommons.usf.edu/etd/494

22 Hidaka M, Wakabayashi I, Takeda Y, Fukuzawa K. Vitamin D₃ derivatives increase soluble CD14 release through ERK1/2 activation and decrease IL-8 production in intestinal epithelial cells. Eur J Pharmacol. 2013 Dec 5;721(1-3):305-12. doi: 10.1016/j.ejphar.2013.09.014. Epub 2013 Sep 20. PMID: 24060240.

23 Ngo DH, Vo TS. An Updated Review on Pharmaceutical Properties of Gamma-Aminobutyric Acid. Molecules. 2019 Jul 24;24(15):2678. doi: 10.3390/molecules24152678. PMID: 31344785; PMCID: PMC6696076.

24 Masoodi M, Peschka M, Schmiedel S, Haddad M, Frye M, Maas C, Lohse A, Huber S, Kirchhof P, Nofer JR, Renné T. Disturbed lipid and amino acid metabolisms in COVID-19 patients. J Mol Med (Berl). 2022 Apr;100(4):555-568. doi: 10.1007/s00109-022-02177-4. Epub 2022 Jan 22. PMID: 35064792; PMCID: PMC8783191.

25 Wang C, Kerckhofs K, Van de Casteele M, Smolders I, Pipeleers D, Ling Z. Glucose inhibits GABA release by pancreatic beta-cells through an increase in GABA shunt activity. Am J Physiol Endocrinol Metab. 2006 Mar;290(3):E494-9. doi: 10.1152/ajpendo.00304.2005. Epub 2005 Oct 25. PMID: 16249254.

26 Deshpande LS, Blair RE, DeLorenzo RJ. Prolonged cannabinoid exposure alters GABA(A) receptor mediated synaptic function in cultured hippocampal neurons. Exp Neurol. 2011 Jun;229(2):264-73. doi: 10.1016/j.expneurol.2011.02.007. Epub 2011 Feb 12. PMID: 21324315; PMCID: PMC3100418.

Curcumin increases GABA.
Curcumol allosterically modulates GABA(A) receptors in a manner distinct from benzodiazepines[27]
Vitamin D deficiency decreases GABA.
Vitamin D deficiency induces the excitation/inhibition brain imbalance and the proinflammatory shift[28]
Gaba is a possible treatment for COVID-19 (Preprint)
GABA administration prevents severe illness and death following coronavirus infection in mice[29]

4. GPNMB (Glycoprotein)
"GPNMB encodes the transmembrane glycoprotein NMB, which could play a role in neurodegenerative disorders[30]."
Covid-19 encodes spike glycoproteins
The SARS-CoV-2 Spike Glycoprotein Biosynthesis, Structure, Function, and Antigenicity: Implications for the Design of Spike-Based Vaccine Immunogens[31]
High Glucose raises spike glycoproteins
Blood glycoprotein levels in diabetes mellitus[32]
Cannabinoids reduce glycoproteins
The effects of cannabinoids on P-glycoprotein transport and expression in multidrug resistant cells[33]
Curcumin reduces glycoproteins
Impact of Curcumin-Induced Changes in P-Glycoprotein and CYP3A Expression on the Pharmacokinetics of Peroral Celiprolol and Midazolam in Rats[34]
Vitamin D reduces glycoproteins
AB0415 The Effect of Vitamin D Supplementation on Antiphospholipid Antibodies Level in Patients with Antiphospholipid Syndrome[35]

Gaba inhibits via the glycoprotein

---

27 Liu YM, Fan HR, Ding J, Huang C, Deng S, Zhu T, Xu TL, Ge WH, Li WG, Li F. Curcumol allosterically modulates GABA(A) receptors in a manner distinct from benzodiazepines. Sci Rep. 2017 Apr 24;7:46654. doi: 10.1038/srep46654. PMID: 28436443; PMCID: PMC5402396.

28 Kasatkina LA, Tarasenko AS, Krupko OO, Kuchmerovska TM, Lisakovska OO, Trikash IO. Vitamin D deficiency induces the excitation/inhibition brain imbalance and the proinflammatory shift. Int J Biochem Cell Biol. 2020 Feb;119:105665. doi: 10.1016/j.biocel.2019.105665. Epub 2019 Dec 9. PMID: 31821883.

29 Tian J, Middleton B, Kaufman DL. GABA administration prevents severe illness and death following coronavirus infection in mice. bioRxiv [Preprint]. 2020 Oct 4:2020.10.04.325423. doi: 10.1101/2020.10.04.325423. Update in: Viruses. 2021 May 23;13(6): PMID: 33024975; PMCID: PMC7536896.

30 Michel Neidhart, Chapter 17 - DNA Methylation in Psychiatric Diseases,
Editor(s): Michel Neidhart, DNA Methylation and Complex Human Disease,
Academic Press, 2016, Pages 289-314, ISBN 9780124201941, https://doi.org/10.1016/B978-0-12-420194-1.00017-8.

31 Duan L, Zheng Q, Zhang H, Niu Y, Lou Y, Wang H. The SARS-CoV-2 Spike Glycoprotein Biosynthesis, Structure, Function, and Antigenicity: Implications for the Design of Spike-Based Vaccine Immunogens. Front Immunol. 2020 Oct 7;11:576622. doi: 10.3389/fimmu.2020.576622. PMID: 33117378; PMCID: PMC7575906.

32 Jonsson A, Wales JK. Blood glycoprotein levels in diabetes mellitus. Diabetologia. 1976 Jul;12(3):245-50. doi: 10.1007/BF00422091. PMID: 60265.

33 Holland ML, Panetta JA, Hoskins JM, Bebawy M, Roufogalis BD, Allen JD, Arnold JC. The effects of cannabinoids on P-glycoprotein transport and expression in multidrug resistant cells. Biochem Pharmacol. 2006 Apr 14;71(8):1146-54. doi: 10.1016/j.bcp.2005.12.033. Epub 2006 Feb 2. PMID: 16458258.

34 Wenxia Zhang, Theresa May Chin Tan and Lee-Yong Lim Drug Metabolism and Disposition January 2007, 35 (1) 110-115; DOI: https://doi.org/10.1124/dmd.106.011072

35 Soroka N, Talako TAB0415 The Effect of Vitamin D Supplementation on Antiphospholipid Antibodies Level in Patients with Antiphospholipid SyndromeAnnals of the Rheumatic Diseases 2016;75:1048.

5. HSP90 AA1 (Heat Shock Protein)

"A generic term for a family of molecular chaperones which play a key role in protein folding and quality control for a range of client proteins. Functional HSP90s operate as dimers, have intrinsic ATPase activity, act in concert with other chaperones (e.g., HSP70) and are regulated by co-chaperones/accessory proteins (e.g., HOP, CDC37). HSP90s interact with more than 100 proteins, including kinases (e.g., Raf-1), nuclear hormone receptors (e.g., oestrogen receptor), transcription factors (e.g., P53), GPCRs (e.g., CB2 receptors) and ion channels (e.g. CFTR). In humans, the HSP90-beta isoform is constitutively expressed (i.e., at baseline), whereas HSP90-alpha isoforms are induced by stress."[37]

Covid-19 uses heat shock protein to infect
Human coronavirus dependency on host heat shock protein 90 reveals an antiviral target [38]

Heat-shock protein causes insulin resistance
Exercise, heat shock proteins and insulin resistance[39]

Cannabinoids reduce expression of heat-shock proteins
Cannabidiol Modulates the Immunophenotype and Inhibits the Activation of the Inflammasome in Human Gingival Mesenchymal Stem Cells (table 3A)[40]

Curcumin: reduces heat-shock protein
Curcumin derivative C212 inhibits Hsp90 and eliminates both growing and quiescent leukemia cells in deep dormancy[41]

Vitamin D: no effect
Vitamin D supplementation and serum heat shock protein 60 levels in patients with coronary heart disease: a randomized clinical trial[42]

HSP limits Gaba release
MaxiK Channel Interactome Reveals its Interaction with GABA Transporter 3 and Heat Shock Protein 60 in the Mammalian Brain - PMC (nih.gov)

6. p38 MAPK (mitogen-activated protein kinase)

"Mitogen activated protein kinase p38 (p38MAPK) is an important intracellular kinase activated by cellular stress that links inflammatory as well as environmental stress to transcription factors [43]."

Covid-19 signals proinflammatory, pro-vasconstrictive, pro-thrombotic activity via p38

36 Jewett BE, Sharma S. Physiology, GABA. [Updated 2021 Jul 26]. In: StatPearls [Internet]. Treasure Island (FL): StatPearls Publishing; 2022 Jan-. Available from: https://www.ncbi.nlm.nih.gov/books/NBK513311/

37 "Hsp90 heat-shock proteins." Segen's Medical Dictionary. 2011. Farlex, Inc. 21 Jul. 2022 https://medical-dictionary.thefreedictionary.com/Hsp90+heat-shock+proteins

38 Li, Cun et al. "Human coronavirus dependency on host heat shock protein 90 reveals an antiviral target." Emerging microbes & infections vol. 9,1 (2020): 2663-2672. doi:10.1080/22221751.2020.1850183

39 Archer, Ashley E et al. "Exercise, heat shock proteins and insulin resistance." Philosophical transactions of the Royal Society of London. Series B, Biological sciences vol. 373,1738 (2018): 20160529. doi:10.1098/rstb.2016.0529

40 Libro R, Scionti D, Diomede F, Marchisio M, Grassi G, Pollastro F, Piattelli A, Bramanti P, Mazzon E, Trubiani O. Cannabidiol Modulates the Immunophenotype and Inhibits the Activation of the Inflammasome in Human Gingival Mesenchymal Stem Cells. Front Physiol. 2016 Nov 24;7:559. doi: 10.3389/fphys.2016.00559. PMID: 27932991; PMCID: PMC5121123.

41 Liu, B., Shen, Y., Huang, H. et al. Curcumin derivative C212 inhibits Hsp90 and eliminates both growing and quiescent leukemia cells in deep dormancy. Cell Commun Signal 18, 159 (2020). https://doi.org/10.1186/s12964-020-00652-4

42 Bahrami, L.S., Sezavar Seyedi Jandaghi, S.H., Janani, L. et al. Vitamin D supplementation and serum heat shock protein 60 levels in patients with coronary heart disease: a randomized clinical trial. Nutr Metab (Lond) 15, 56 (2018). https://doi.org/10.1186/s12986-018-0292-9

43 From: Handbook of Cell Signaling (Second Edition), 2010

p38 MAPK inhibition: A promising therapeutic approach for COVID-19[44]

High Glucose activates p38

Glucose or diabetes activates p38 mitogen-activanhted protein kinase via different pathways[45]

Cannabinoids suppress p38

Immune Responses Regulated by Cannabidiol[46]

Curcumin suppresses p38

<u>*Curcumin suppress inflammatory response in traumatic brain injury via p38/MAPK signaling pathway*</u> *[47]*

Vitamin D suppresses p38

Inhibition of p38 by Vitamin D Reduces Interleukin-6 Production in Normal Prostate Cells via Mitogen-Activated Protein Kinase Phosphatase 5: Implications for Prostate Cancer Prevention by Vitamin D[48]

Inefficient Gaba signaling system increases cytokine signaling system via p38 MARK

Does gamma-aminobutyric acid (GABA) influence the development of chronic inflammation in rheumatoid arthritis?[49]

7. TMPRSS2 (transmembrane serine protease 2)

"TMPRSS2 is an endothelial cell surface protein that is involved in the viral entry and spread of coronaviruses including severe acute respiratory syndrome coronavirus 2 (SARS-CoV-2) – the virus that causes COVID19. Blocking TMPRSS2 could potentially be an effective clinical therapy for COVID-19." (<u>What is</u> <u>TMPRSS2? News Medical Life Sciences</u>)

A variant in TMPRSS2 is associated with decreased disease severity in COVID-19[50]

Covid-19 infects via TMPRSS2

<u>*Altered TMPRSS2 usage by SARS-CoV-2 Omicron impacts tropism and fusogenicity*</u>*[51]*

Diabetes increases TMPRSS2 expression

Glycated ACE2 receptor in diabetes: open door for SARS-COV-2 entry in cardiomyocyte[52]

Some Cannabinoid extracts down-regulate TMPRSS2

In search of preventive strategies: novel high-CBD Cannabis sativa extracts modulate ACE2 expression in COVID-19 gateway tissues[53]

44 Grimes, Joseph M, and Kevin V Grimes. "p38 MAPK inhibition: A promising therapeutic approach for COVID-19." Journal of molecular and cellular cardiology vol. 144 (2020): 63-65. doi:10.1016/j.yjmcc.2020.05.007

45 Igarashi, M et al. "Glucose or diabetes activates p38 mitogen-activated protein kinase via different pathways." The Journal of clinical investigation vol. 103,2 (1999): 185-95. doi:10.1172/JCI3326

46 James M. Nichols and Barbara L.F. Kaplan.Cannabis and Cannabinoid Research.Mar 2020.12 31.http://doi.org/10.1089/can.2018.0073

47 Li, G., Duan, L., Yang, F., Yang, L., Deng, Y., Yu, Y., Xu, Y., & Zhang, Y. (2022). Curcumin suppress inflammatory response in traumatic brain injury via p38/MAPK signaling pathway. Phytotherapy Research, 1– 12. https://doi.org/10.1002/ptr.7391

48 Nonn L, Peng L, Feldman D, Peehl DM. Inhibition of p38 by vitamin D reduces interleukin-6 production in normal prostate cells via mitogen-activated protein kinase phosphatase 5: implications for prostate cancer prevention by vitamin D. Cancer Res. 2006 Apr 15;66(8):4516-24. doi: 10.1158/0008-5472.CAN-05-3796. PMID: 16618780.

49 Kelley, J.M., Hughes, L.B. & Bridges, S.L. Does gamma-aminobutyric acid (GABA) influence the development of chronic inflammation in rheumatoid arthritis?. J Neuroinflammation 5, 1 (2008). https://doi.org/10.1186/1742-2094-5-1

50 Ravikanth V, Sasikala M, Naveen V, Latha SS, Parsa KVL, Vijayasarathy K, Amanchy R, Avanthi S, Govardhan B, Rakesh K, Kumari DS, Srikaran B, Rao GV, Reddy DN. A variant in TMPRSS2 is associated with decreased disease severity in COVID-19. Meta Gene. 2021 Sep;29:100930. doi: 10.1016/j.mgene.2021.100930. Epub 2021 May 28. PMID: 34075330; PMCID: PMC8161869.

51 Meng, B., Abdullahi, A., Ferreira, I.A.T.M. et al. Altered TMPRSS2 usage by SARS-CoV-2 Omicron impacts tropism and fusogenicity. Nature (2022). https://doi.org/10.1038/s41586-022-04474-x

52 D'Onofrio, N., Scisciola, L., Sardu, C. et al. Glycated ACE2 receptor in diabetes: open door for SARS-COV-2 entry in cardiomyocyte. Cardiovasc Diabetol 20, 99 (2021). https://doi.org/10.1186/s12933-021-01286-7

53 Wang B, Kovalchuk A, Li D, Rodriguez-Juarez R, Ilnytskyy Y, Kovalchuk I, Kovalchuk O. In search of preventive strategies: novel high-CBD Cannabis sativa extracts modulate ACE2 expression in COVID-19 gateway tissues. Aging

Curcumin decreases activity of TMPRSS2

Phenolic compounds disrupt spike-mediated receptor-binding and entry of SARS-CoV-2 pseudo-virions[54]

Vitamin D reduces TMPRSS2

Synergy of melanin and vitamin-D may play a fundamental role in preventing SARS-CoV-2 infections and halt COVID-19 by inactivating furin protease[55]

Gaba: no data found

8. TLR (Toll-like receptor, TLR2-TLR9)

"Toll like receptors (TLR) are key molecules expressed by innate immune cells that enable them to detect pathogen associated molecular patterns and recognize pathogens to mount immune responses."[56]

Covid-19 uses TLR to infect

Role of Toll-like receptors in the pathogenesis of COVID-19[57]

High Glucose induces TLR

High glucose induces toll-like receptor expression in human monocytes: mechanism of activation[58]

Cannabinoids use TLR to control inflammation

Interaction between Cannabinoid System and Toll-Like Receptors Controls Inflammation[59]

Curcumin reduces TLR expression

Impact of curcumin on toll-like receptors[60]

Curcumin decreases toll-like receptor-2 gene expression and function in human monocytes and neutrophils[61]

Vitamin D might have immunomodulatory effects via TLR

Vitamin D and toll like receptors[62]

Vitamin D up-regulates TLR

Toll-like receptor triggering of a vitamin D-mediated human antimicrobial response[63]

(Albany NY). 2020 Nov 22;12(22):22425-22444. doi: 10.18632/aging.202225. Epub 2020 Nov 22. PMID: 33221759; PMCID: PMC7746344.

54 Goc A, Sumera W, Rath M, Niedzwiecki A. Phenolic compounds disrupt spike-mediated receptor-binding and entry of SARS-CoV-2 pseudo-virions. PLoS One. 2021 Jun 17;16(6):e0253489. doi: 10.1371/journal.pone.0253489. PMID: 34138966; PMCID: PMC8211150.

55 Paria, K., Paul, D., Chowdhury, T. et al. Synergy of melanin and vitamin-D may play a fundamental role in preventing SARS-CoV-2 infections and halt COVID-19 by inactivating furin protease. transl med commun 5, 21 (2020). https://doi.org/10.1186/s41231-020-00073-y

56 From: Advances in Immunology, 2020

57 Khanmohammadi S, Rezaei N. Role of Toll-like receptors in the pathogenesis of COVID-19. J Med Virol. 2021 May;93(5):2735-2739. doi: 10.1002/jmv.26826. Epub 2021 Feb 9. PMID: 33506952; PMCID: PMC8014260.

58 Dasu MR, Devaraj S, Zhao L, Hwang DH, Jialal I. High glucose induces toll-like receptor expression in human monocytes: mechanism of activation. Diabetes. 2008 Nov;57(11):3090-8. doi: 10.2337/db08-0564. Epub 2008 Jul 23. PMID: 18650365; PMCID: PMC2570406.

59 McCoy KL. Interaction between Cannabinoid System and Toll-Like Receptors Controls Inflammation. Mediators Inflamm. 2016;2016:5831315. doi: 10.1155/2016/5831315. Epub 2016 Aug 11. PMID: 27597805; PMCID: PMC4997072.

60 Boozari M, Butler AE, Sahebkar A. Impact of curcumin on toll-like receptors. J Cell Physiol. 2019 Aug;234(8):12471-12482. doi: 10.1002/jcp.28103. Epub 2019 Jan 8. PMID: 30623441.

61 Shuto T, Ono T, Ohira Y, Shimasaki S, Mizunoe S, Watanabe K, Suico MA, Koga T, Sato T, Morino S, Sato K, Kai H. Curcumin decreases toll-like receptor-2 gene expression and function in human monocytes and neutrophils. Biochem Biophys Res Commun. 2010 Aug 6;398(4):647-52. doi: 10.1016/j.bbrc.2010.06.126. Epub 2010 Jul 3. PMID: 20599422.

62 Arababadi MK, Nosratabadi R, Asadikaram G. Vitamin D and toll like receptors. Life Sci. 2018 Jun 15;203:105-111. doi: 10.1016/j.lfs.2018.03.040. Epub 2018 Mar 27. PMID: 29596922.

63 Liu PT, Stenger S, Li H, Wenzel L, Tan BH, Krutzik SR, Ochoa MT, Schauber J, Wu K, Meinken C, Kamen DL, Wagner M, Bals R, Steinmeyer A, Zügel U, Gallo RL, Eisenberg D, Hewison M, Hollis BW, Adams JS, Bloom BR, Modlin RL. Toll-like receptor triggering of a vitamin D-mediated human antimicrobial response. Science. 2006 Mar 24;311(5768):1770-3. doi: 10.1126/science.1123933. Epub 2006 Feb 23. PMID: 16497887.

Gaba reduces inflammation via TLR
Gama-aminobutyric acid (GABA) alleviates hepatic inflammation via GABA receptors/TLR4/NF-κB pathways in growing-finishing pigs generated by super-multiparous sows[64]

CYTOKINES/CHEMOKINES

Cytokines/chemokines

"Cytokines and chemokines are redundant secreted proteins with growth, differentiation, and activation functions that regulate and determine the nature of immune responses and control immune cell trafficking and the cellular arrangement of immune organs. Which cytokines are produced in response to an immune insult determines initially whether an immune response develops and subsequently whether that response is cytotoxic, humoral, cell-mediated, or allergic. A cascade of responses can be seen in response to cytokines, and often several cytokines are required to synergize to express optimal function. An additional confounding variable in dissecting cytokine function is that each cytokine may have a completely different function, depending on the cellular source, target, and, most important, specific phase of the immune response during which it is presented. Numerous cytokines have both proinflammatory and anti-inflammatory potential; which activity is observed depends on the immune cells present and their state of responsiveness to the cytokine."[65]

9. CCL2 (CC chemokine or monocyte chemoattractant protein-1 (MCP-1). "CCL2 is the best-known CC chemokine, otherwise called as monocyte chemoattractant protein-1 (MCP-1), which attracts monocytes expressing CCR2 receptor in the circulatory system helping them to enter the encompassing injured and inflamed tissues where they transform into tissue macrophages.[66]"
Covid-19 increases CCL2.
Longitudinal profiling of respiratory and systemic immune responses reveals myeloid cell-driven lung inflammation in severe COVID-19[67]
IP-10 and MCP-1 as biomarkers associated with disease severity of COVID-19[68]
High glucose increases CCL2 (MCP-2)
Monocyte Chemoattractant Protein 1 (MCP-1) in Obesity and Diabetes[69]

Fasting decreases CCL2 (MCP-2)

64 Zhang S, Zhao J, Hu J, He H, Wei Y, Ji L, Ma X. Gama-aminobutyric acid (GABA) alleviates hepatic inflammation via GABA receptors/TLR4/NF-κB pathways in growing-finishing pigs generated by super-multiparous sows. Anim Nutr. 2022 Feb 17;9:280-290. doi: 10.1016/j.aninu.2022.02.001. PMID: 35600552; PMCID: PMC9092368.

65 Borish LC, Steinke JW. 2. Cytokines and chemokines. J Allergy Clin Immunol. 2003 Feb;111(2 Suppl):S460-75. doi: 10.1067/mai.2003.108. PMID: 12592293.

66 Singhal, Gaurav & Baune, Bernhard. (2018). Do Chemokines Have a Role in the Pathophysiology of Depression?. 10.1016/B978-0-12-811073-7.00008-8.

67 Peter A. Szabo, Pranay Dogra, Joshua I. Gray, Steven B. Wells, Thomas J. Connors, Stuart P. Weisberg, Izabela Krupska, Rei Matsumoto, Maya M.L. Poon, Emma Idzikowski, Sinead E. Morris, Chloé Pasin, Andrew J. Yates, Amy Ku, Michael Chait, Julia Davis-Porada, Xinzheng V. Guo, Jing Zhou, Matthew Steinle, Sean Mackay, Anjali Saqi, Matthew R. Baldwin, Peter A. Sims, Donna L. Farber, Longitudinal profiling of respiratory and systemic immune responses reveals myeloid cell-driven lung inflammation in severe COVID-19, Immunity, Volume 54, Issue 4, 2021, Pages 797-814.e6, ISSN 1074-7613, https://doi.org/10.1016/j.immuni.2021.03.005.

68 Chen, Y., Wang, J., Liu, C. et al. IP-10 and MCP-1 as biomarkers associated with disease severity of COVID-19. Mol Med 26, 97 (2020). https://doi.org/10.1186/s10020-020-00230-x

69 Panee, Jun. "Monocyte Chemoattractant Protein 1 (MCP-1) in obesity and diabetes." Cytokine vol. 60,1 (2012): 1-12. doi:10.1016/j.cyto.2012.06.018

Intermittent Fasting Improves Glucose Tolerance and Promotes Adipose Tissue Remodeling in Male Mice Fed a High-Fat Diet[70]

Cannabinoids decrease CCL2 (MCP-2)

THC: *Δ9-Tetrahydrocannabinol Suppresses Monocyte-Mediated Astrocyte Production of Monocyte Chemoattractant Protein 1 and Interleukin-6 in a Toll-Like Receptor 7–Stimulated Human Coculture*[71]

CBD: *Cannabis compounds exhibit anti-inflammatory activity in vitro in COVID-19-related inflammation in lung epithelial cells and pro-inflammatory activity in macrophages*[72]

Curcumin Decreases CCL2

Curcumin blocks CCL2-induced adhesion, motility and invasion, in part, through down-regulation of CCL2 expression and proteolytic activity[73]

Curcumin as a natural regulator of monocyte chemoattractant protein-1[74]

Vitamin D Decreases CCL2.

Vitamin D Limits Chemokine Expression in Adipocytes and Macrophage Migration In Vitro and in Male Mice[75]

Effect of Vitamin D3 on Monocyte Chemoattractant Protein 1 Production in Monocytes and Macrophages[76]

Increasing CCL2 (MCP1) decreases GABA

GABA administration prevents severe illness and death following coronavirus infection in mice[77]

Anti-inflammatory effects of the GABA(B) receptor agonist baclofen in allergic contact dermatitis[78]

10. CCL3/ MIP-a (macrophage inflammatory protein-1 α and macrophage inflammatory protein 1-alpha)

"CCL3 is expressed constitutively in the bone marrow, including by osteoblasts, and is induced during inflammation. Bacterial toxins, viral infections, TNFα, IFN-γ, IL-1β, and IL-6 are some of the stimuli that induce the expression of CCL3 and/or CCL4 in vitro from multiple cell types including monocytes/macrophages, DCs, and epithelial cells. In addition, IL-10, IL-

70 Endocrinology, Volume 160, Issue 1, January 2019, Pages 169–180

71 Rizzo MD, Crawford RB, Bach A, Sermet S, Amalfitano A, Kaminski NE. Δ9-Tetrahydrocannabinol Suppresses Monocyte-Mediated Astrocyte Production of Monocyte Chemoattractant Protein 1 and Interleukin-6 in a Toll-Like Receptor 7-Stimulated Human Coculture. J Pharmacol Exp Ther. 2019 Oct;371(1):191-201. doi: 10.1124/jpet.119.260661. Epub 2019 Aug 5. PMID: 31383729; PMCID: PMC7184191.

72 Anil SM, Shalev N, Vinayaka AC, Nadarajan S, Namdar D, Belausov E, Shoval I, Mani KA, Mechrez G, Koltai H. Cannabis compounds exhibit anti-inflammatory activity in vitro in COVID-19-related inflammation in lung epithelial cells and pro-inflammatory activity in macrophages. Sci Rep. 2021 Jan 14;11(1):1462. doi: 10.1038/s41598-021-81049-2. PMID: 33446817; PMCID: PMC7809280.

73 Herman JG, Stadelman HL, Roselli CE. Curcumin blocks CCL2-induced adhesion, motility and invasion, in part, through down-regulation of CCL2 expression and proteolytic activity. Int J Oncol. 2009 May;34(5):1319-27. PMID: 19360344; PMCID: PMC2683974.

74 Karimian MS, Pirro M, Majeed M, Sahebkar A. Curcumin as a natural regulator of monocyte chemoattractant protein-1. Cytokine Growth Factor Rev. 2017 Feb;33:55-63. doi: 10.1016/j.cytogfr.2016.10.001. Epub 2016 Oct 8. PMID: 27743775.

75 Esma Karkeni, Julie Marcotorchino, Franck Tourniaire, Julien Astier, Franck Peiretti, Patrice Darmon, Jean-François Landrier, Vitamin D Limits Chemokine Expression in Adipocytes and Macrophage Migration In Vitro and in Male Mice, Endocrinology, Volume 156, Issue 5, 1 May 2015, Pages 1782–1793, https://doi.org/10.1210/en.2014-1647

76 Wang, Yi-Chen et al. "Effect of Vitamin D3 on Monocyte Chemoattractant Protein 1 Production in Monocytes and Macrophages." Acta Cardiologica Sinica vol. 30,2 (2014): 144-50.

77 Tian J, Middleton B, Kaufman DL. GABA administration prevents severe illness and death following coronavirus infection in mice. bioRxiv [Preprint]. 2020 Oct 4:2020.10.04.325423. doi: 10.1101/2020.10.04.325423. Update in: Viruses. 2021 May 23;13(6): PMID: 33024975; PMCID: PMC7536896.

78 Duthey B, Hübner A, Diehl S, Boehncke S, Pfeffer J, Boehncke WH. Anti-inflammatory effects of the GABA(B) receptor agonist baclofen in allergic contact dermatitis. Exp Dermatol. 2010 Jul 1;19(7):661-6. doi: 10.1111/j.1600-0625.2010.01076.x. Epub 2010 Feb 25. PMID: 20201957.

4, and transforming growth factor-β attenuate the inflammation-induced expression of these two chemokines."[79]

"Macrophage inflammatory protein-1α (MIP-1α) and MIP-1β are distinct but highly homologous CC chemokines produced by a variety of host cells in response to various external stimuli and share affinity for CCR5. To better elucidate the role of these CC chemokines in adaptive immunity, we have characterized the affects of MIP-1α and MIP-1β on cellular and humoral immune responses. MIP-1α stimulated strong antigen (Ag)–specific serum immunoglobulin G (IgG) and IgM responses, while MIP-1β promoted lower IgG and IgM but higher serum IgA and IgE antibody (Ab) responses. MIP-1α elevated Ag-specific IgG1 and IgG2b followed by IgG2a and IgG3 subclass responses, while MIP-1β only stimulated IgG1 and IgG2b subclasses. Correspondingly, MIP-1β produced higher titers of Ag-specific mucosal secretory IgA Ab levels when compared with MIP-1α."[80]

Covid-19 raises CCL3 (MIP-1a)
Cytokine Profiles Associated With Worse Prognosis in a Hospitalized Peruvian COVID-19 Cohort[81]

Glucose raises CCL3 (MIP-1a)
Glucose-induced expression of MIP-1 genes requires O-GlcNAc transferase in monocytes[82]

Cannabinoids inhibit CCL3 (MIP-1a)
Heavy Cannabis Use Associated With Reduction in Activated and Inflammatory Immune Cell Frequencies in Antiretroviral Therapy–Treated Human Immunodeficiency Virus–Infected Individuals[83]

Curcumin inhibits CCL3 (MIP-1a)
Curcumin inhibition of inflammatory cytokine production by human peripheral blood monocytes and alveolar macrophages[84]

Vitamin D suppresses CCL3 (MIP-1a)
Effect of Vitamin D3 on Monocyte Chemoattractant Protein 1 Production in Monocytes and Macrophages[85]

Gaba: no data found

_____

79 Ronald L. Rabin, CC, C, and CX3C Chemokines, Editor(s): Helen L. Henry, Anthony W. Norman, Encyclopedia of Hormones, Academic Press, 2003, Pages 255-263, ISBN 9780123411037, https://doi.org/10.1016/B0-12-341103-3/00044-9

80 James W. Lillard, Udai P. Singh, Prosper N. Boyaka, Shailesh Singh, Dennis D. Taub, Jerry R. McGhee; MIP-1α and MIP-1β differentially mediate mucosal and systemic adaptive immunity. Blood 2003; 101 (3): 807–814. doi: https://doi.org/10.1182/blood-2002-07-2305

81 Pons Maria J., YmaÃ±a Barbara, Mayanga-Herrera Ana, SÃ¡enz Yolanda, Alvarez-Erviti Lydia, Tapia-Rojas Salyoc, Gamarra Roxana, Blanco Amanda B., Moncunill Gemma, Ugarte-Gil Manuel F. Cytokine Profiles Associated With Worse Prognosis in a Hospitalized Peruvian COVID-19 Cohort. Frontiers in Immunology. Volume 12, 2021. https://www.frontiersin.org/article/10.3389/fimmu.2021.700921. DOI=10.3389/fimmu.2021.700921. ISSN=1664-3224

82 Chikanishi T, Fujiki R, Hashiba W, Sekine H, Yokoyama A, Kato S. Glucose-induced expression of MIP-1 genes requires O-GlcNAc transferase in monocytes. Biochem Biophys Res Commun. 2010 Apr 16;394(4):865-70. doi: 10.1016/j.bbrc.2010.02.167. Epub 2010 Mar 2. PMID: 20206135.

83 Manuzak, Jennifer & Gott, Toni & Kirkwood, Jay & Coronado, Ernesto & Hensley-McBain, Tiffany & Miller, Charlene & Cheu, Ryan & Collier, Ann & Funderburg, Nicholas & Martin, Jeffery & Wu, Michael & Isoherranen, Nina & Hunt, Peter & Klatt, Nichole. (2018). Heavy Cannabis Use Associated With Reduction in Activated and Inflammatory Immune Cell Frequencies in Antiretroviral Therapy-Treated Human Immunodeficiency Virus-Infected Individuals. Clinical infectious diseases : an official publication of the Infectious Diseases Society of America. 66. 10.1093/cid/cix1116.

84 Abe Y, Hashimoto S, Horie T. Curcumin inhibition of inflammatory cytokine production by human peripheral blood monocytes and alveolar macrophages. Pharmacol Res. 1999 Jan;39(1):41-7. doi: 10.1006/phrs.1998.0404. PMID: 10051376.

85 Jennifer A Manuzak, Toni M Gott, Jay S Kirkwood, Ernesto Coronado, Tiffany Hensley-McBain, Charlene Miller, Ryan K Cheu, Ann C Collier, Nicholas T Funderburg, Jeffery N Martin, Michael C Wu, Nina Isoherranen, Peter W Hunt, Nichole R Klatt, Heavy Cannabis Use Associated With Reduction in Activated and Inflammatory Immune Cell Frequencies in Antiretroviral Therapy–Treated Human Immunodeficiency Virus–Infected Individuals, Clinical Infectious Diseases, Volume 66, Issue 12, 15 June 2018, Pages 1872–1882, https://doi.org/10.1093/cid/cix1116

11. CCL4 (MIP-1b) CCR5 receptor

"CCL4, a CC chemokine, previously known as macrophage inflammatory protein (MIP)-1β, has diverse effects on various types of immune and nonimmune cells by the virtue of its interaction with its specific receptor, CCR5, in collaboration with related but distinct CC chemokines such as CCL3 and CCL5, which can also bind CCR5. Several lines of evidence indicate that CCL4 can promote tumor development and progression by recruiting regulatory T cells and pro-tumorigenic macrophages, and acting on other resident cells present in the tumor microenvironment, such as fibroblasts and endothelial cells, to facilitate their pro-tumorigenic capacities." (***CCL4 Signaling in the Tumor Microenvironment***)[86]

Covid-19 increases CCL4 (MIP-1b) levels
MIP-1a and MIP-1b in serum as potential markers of the severe course COVID-19[87]

High Glucose increases CCL4 (MIP-1b) levels
MCP-1 and MIP-2 expression and production in BB diabetic rat: effect of chronic hypoxia[88]

Cannabinoids lower CCL4 (MIP-1b)
Heavy Cannabis Use Associated with Reduction in Activated and Inflammatory Immune Cell Frequencies in Antiretroviral Therapy-Treated Human Immunodeficiency Virus-Infected Individuals[89]

Curcumin lowers CCL4 (MIP-1b)
Curcumin inhibition of inflammatory cytokine production by human peripheral blood monocytes and alveolar macrophages[90]

Vitamin D lowers CCL4 (MIP-1b)
Effect of Vitamin D3 on Monocyte Chemoattractant Protein 1 Production in Monocytes and Macrophages[91]

Gaba: no data found

12. CCL5 (RANTES)

"CCR1, CCR3, and CCR5 all function as receptors for CCL5. Thus, CCL5 produces signals in monocytes, macrophages, T-cell subsets, DCs, eosinophils, basophils, and microglia. In addition to its chemoattractant activity, CCL5 stimulates eosinophils to secrete eosinophil cationic protein and stimulates basophils to release histamine. Mononuclear cells in CCL5 KO mice migrate less to sites of cutaneous hypersensitivity and T cells from these mice proliferate less in vitro in response to mitogens and specific antigens. The effects of CCL5 overexpression in animal models or challenge in humans vary with the anatomic site and type of challenge. Intratracheal challenge of Sprague–Dawley rats with CCL5-expressing adenovirus showed enhanced monocyte recruitment to the lung by approximately

86 Mukaida N, Sasaki SI, Baba T. CCL4 Signaling in the Tumor Microenvironment. Adv Exp Med Biol. 2020;1231:23-32. doi: 10.1007/978-3-030-36667-4_3. PMID: 32060843.

87 A. Grishaeva, Z. Ponezheva, M. Chanyshev, A. Ploskireva, D. Usenko, N. Tsvetkova, K. Omarova, N. Pshenichnaya, MIP-1a and MIP-1b in serum as potential markers of the severe course COVID-19, International Journal of Infectious Diseases, Volume 116, Supplement, 2022, Page S44, ISSN 1201-9712, https://doi.org/10.1016/j.ijid.2021.12.105.

88 Marisa C, Lucci I, Di Giulio C, Bianchi G, Grilli A, Patruno A, Reale M. MCP-1 and MIP-2 expression and production in BB diabetic rat: effect of chronic hypoxia. Mol Cell Biochem. 2005 Aug;276(1-2):105-11. doi: 10.1007/s11010-005-3556-4. PMID: 16132691.

89 Jennifer A Manuzak, Toni M Gott, Jay S Kirkwood, Ernesto Coronado, Tiffany Hensley-McBain, Charlene Miller, Ryan K Cheu, Ann C Collier, Nicholas T Funderburg, Jeffery N Martin, Michael C Wu, Nina Isoherranen, Peter W Hunt, Nichole R Klatt, Heavy Cannabis Use Associated With Reduction in Activated and Inflammatory Immune Cell Frequencies in Antiretroviral Therapy–Treated Human Immunodeficiency Virus–Infected Individuals, Clinical Infectious Diseases, Volume 66, Issue 12, 15 June 2018, Pages 1872–1882, https://doi.org/10.1093/cid/cix1116

90 Abe Y, Hashimoto S, Horie T. Curcumin inhibition of inflammatory cytokine production by human peripheral blood monocytes and alveolar macrophages. Pharmacol Res. 1999 Jan;39(1):41-7. doi: 10.1006/phrs.1998.0404. PMID: 10051376.

91 Wang, Yi-Chen et al. "Effect of Vitamin D3 on Monocyte Chemoattractant Protein 1 Production in Monocytes and Macrophages." Acta Cardiologica Sinica vol. 30,2 (2014): 144-50.

50-fold, although CCL5 challenge to nasal mucosa of allergic patients induced eosinophil influx. CCL5 is expressed in lungs of patients with chronic eosinophilic pneumonia, suggesting that CCL5 has a role in eosinophil-induced pathology and that CCL5 blockade may be beneficial in treatment of atopic diseases, including asthma."[92]

Disruption of CCL5 (RANTES) reduces coronavirus propagation
Disruption of the CCL5/RANTES-CCR5 Pathway Restores Immune Homeostasis and Reduces Plasma Viral Load in Critical COVID-19[93]

CCL5 (RANTES) disrupts glucose insulin release
RANTES (CCL5) reduces glucose-dependent secretion of glucagon-like peptides 1 and 2 and impairs glucose-induced insulin secretion in mice[94]

Cannabinoids inhibit CCL5 (RANTES).
The cannabinoid delta-9-tetrahydrocannabinol mediates inhibition of macrophage chemotaxis to RANTES/CCL5: linkage to the CB2 receptor[95]
Δ9 Tetrahydrocannabinol and cannabidiol alter cytokine production by human immune cells[96]

Curcumin lowers serum levels of CCL5 (RANTES)
Effect of curcumin supplementation on serum expression of select cytokines and chemokines in a female rat model of nonalcoholic steatohepatitis[97]

Vitamin D decreases CCL5 (RANTES)
Vitamin D analogs decrease in vitro secretion of RANTES and enhance the effect of budesonide[98]

Gaba inhibits CCL5 (RANTES)
Anti-inflammatory effects of the GABA(B) receptor agonist baclofen in allergic contact dermatitis[99]

13. CCL7 (C-C motif chemokine ligand) MCP-3
"A gene on chromosome 17q11.2-q12 that encodes monocyte chemotactic protein 3 (MCP-3), a secreted chemokine that attracts macrophages during inflammation and metastasis. MCP-3/CCL7 is a member of the C-C subfamily of chemokines, which have two adjacent cysteine residues, and is a

---

92 Ronald L. Rabin, in Encyclopedia of Hormones, 2003

93 Disruption of the CCL5/RANTES-CCR5 Pathway Restores Immune Homeostasis and Reduces Plasma Viral Load in Critical COVID-19 Bruce K. Patterson, Harish Seethamraju, Kush Dhody, Michael J. Corley, Kazem Kazempour, Jay Lalezari, Alina P.S. Pang, Christopher Sugai, Edgar B. Francisco, Amruta Pise, Hallison Rodrigues, Mathew Ryou, Helen L. Wu, Gabriela M. Webb, Byung S. Park, Scott Kelly, Nader Pourhassan, Alena Lelic, Lama Kdouh, Monica Herrera, Eric Hall, Enver Aklin, Lishomwa C. Ndhlovu, Jonah B. Sacha
   medRxiv 2020.05.02.20084673; doi: https://doi.org/10.1101/2020.05.02.20084673

94 RANTES (CCL5) reduces glucose-dependent secretion of glucagon-like peptides 1 and 2 and impairs glucose-induced insulin secretion in mice Ramona Pais, Tamara Zietek, Hans Hauner, Hannelore Daniel, and Thomas Skurk
   American Journal of Physiology-Gastrointestinal and Liver Physiology 2014 307:3, G330-G337

95vRaborn ES, Marciano-Cabral F, Buckley NE, Martin BR, Cabral GA. The cannabinoid delta-9-tetrahydrocannabinol mediates inhibition of macrophage chemotaxis to RANTES/CCL5: linkage to the CB2 receptor. J Neuroimmune Pharmacol. 2008 Jun;3(2):117-29. doi: 10.1007/s11481-007-9077-z. Epub 2007 Jul 11. PMID: 18247131; PMCID: PMC2677557.

96 Maya D Srivastava, B.I.S Srivastava, B Brouhard, Tetrahydrocannabinol and cannabidiol alter cytokine production by human immune cells, Immunopharmacology, Volume 40, Issue 3, 1998, Pages 179-185, ISSN 0162-3109, https://doi.org/10.1016/S0162-3109(98)00041-1.

97 Pickich, M.B., Hargrove, M.W., Phillips, C.N. et al. Effect of curcumin supplementation on serum expression of select cytokines and chemokines in a female rat model of nonalcoholic steatohepatitis. BMC Res Notes 12, 496 (2019). https://doi.org/10.1186/s13104-019-4540-

98 M Fraczek, B Rostkowska-Nadolska, D Kusmierz, A Zielinska, J Rok, E Sliupkas-Dyrda, A Grzanka, T Krecicki, M Latocha, Vitamin D analogs decrease in vitro secretion of RANTES and enhance the effect of budesonide, Advances in Medical Sciences, Volume 57, Issue 2, 2012, Pages 290-295, ISSN 1896-1126, https://doi.org/10.2478/v10039-012-0043-5.

99 Duthey B, Hübner A, Diehl S, Boehncke S, Pfeffer J, Boehncke WH. Anti-inflammatory effects of the GABA(B) receptor agonist baclofen in allergic contact dermatitis. Exp Dermatol. 2010 Jul 1;19(7):661-6. doi: 10.1111/j.1600-0625.2010.01076.x. Epub 2010 Feb 25. PMID: 20201957.

ligand for CCR1, CCR2 and CCR3. It is an in vivo substrate of matrix metalloproteinase 2, an enzyme that degrades the extracellular matrix."[100]

Covid-19 releases CCL7 (MCP-3)
Chemokines and chemokine receptors during COVID-19 infection[101]

Sucrose binds to CCL7 (MCP-3)
Potential inhibitors of chemokine function: analysis of noncovalent complexes of CC chemokine and small polyanionic molecules by ESI FT-ICR mass spectrometry[102]

Cannabinoids reduce CCL7 (MCP-3)
Cannabis compounds exhibit anti-inflammatory activity in vitro in COVID-19-related inflammation in lung epithelial cells and pro-inflammatory activity in macrophages[103]

Curcumin inhibits CCL7 (MCP-3)
Anti-inflammatory effects of curcumin in acute lung injury: In vivo and in vitro experimental model studies[104]

Vitamin D lowers CCL7 (MCP-3)
Optimal vitamin D plasma levels are associated with lower bacterial DNA translocation in HIV/hepatitis c virus coinfected patients[105]
Gaba: no data found

14. CCL8 (MCP-2)
"MCPs stimulate the directed migration or chemotaxis (and activation) of leukocytes into sites of inflammation. All MCPs except CCL8 bind to CCR2, which is expressed on monocytes and macrophages, T cells, B cells, dendritic cells, basophils, mast cells, NK cells and neutrophils. CCL2, CCL8 and CCL7 bind to CCR1, which is expressed by monocytes, T cells, DCs, and eosinophils. CCL8, CCL7 and CCL13 bind to CCR3, which is expressed predominantly by eosinophils, basophils, and Th2-polarized CD4+ T cells. CCL8 can also bind CCR5, which is expressed by Th1-polarized CD4+ T cells and effector CD8+ T cells, monocytes, macrophages, and DCs. Arguably the archetypal MCP is CCL2 (MCP-1) and therefore most research has focussed on this chemokine in relation to function and disease."[106]

Anti CCL8 (MCP-2) antibodies have been proposed for Covid-19
Technology - Anti-CCL8 Antibodies for COVID-19 and Other Immune Related Conditions (sc.edu)

Glucose-dependent insulinotropic peptide (GIP) reduces CCL8 (MCP-2)

100 "CCL7." Segen's Medical Dictionary. 2011. Farlex, Inc. 21 Jul. 2022 https://medical-dictionary.thefreedictionary.com/CCL7

101 Khalil BA, Elemam NM, Maghazachi AA. Chemokines and chemokine receptors during COVID-19 infection. Comput Struct Biotechnol J. 2021;19:976-988. doi: 10.1016/j.csbj.2021.01.034. Epub 2021 Jan 27. PMID: 33558827; PMCID: PMC7859556.

102 Yu Y, Sweeney MD, Saad OM, Leary JA. Potential inhibitors of chemokine function: analysis of noncovalent complexes of CC chemokine and small polyanionic molecules by ESI FT-ICR mass spectrometry. J Am Soc Mass Spectrom. 2006 Apr;17(4):524-535. doi: 10.1016/j.jasms.2005.12.008. Epub 2006 Feb 28. PMID: 16503157.

103 Anil, S.M., Shalev, N., Vinayaka, A.C. et al. Cannabis compounds exhibit anti-inflammatory activity in vitro in COVID-19-related inflammation in lung epithelial cells and pro-inflammatory activity in macrophages. Sci Rep 11, 1462 (2021). https://doi.org/10.1038/s41598-021-81049-2

104 Wang Y, Wang Y, Cai N, Xu T, He F. Anti-inflammatory effects of curcumin in acute lung injury: In vivo and in vitro experimental model studies. Int Immunopharmacol. 2021 Jul;96:107600. doi: 10.1016/j.intimp.2021.107600. Epub 2021 Mar 30. PMID: 33798807.

105 García-Álvarez M, Berenguer J, Jiménez-Sousa MÁ, Vázquez-Morón S, Carrero A, Gutiérrez-Rivas M, Aldámiz-Echevarría T, López JC, García-Broncano P, Resino S. Optimal vitamin D plasma levels are associated with lower bacterial DNA translocation in HIV/hepatitis c virus coinfected patients. AIDS. 2016 Apr 24;30(7):1069-74. doi: 10.1097/QAD.0000000000001007. PMID: 27032111.

106 Andrew Williams, in Encyclopedia of Respiratory Medicine(Second Edition), 2022

Long-acting glucose-dependent insulinotropic polypeptide ameliorates obesity-induced adipose tissue inflammation[107]

Cannabinoids reduce CCL8 (MCP-2)

Anti-inflammatory activity of topical THC in DNFB-mediated mouse allergic contact dermatitis independent of CB1 and CB2 receptors[108]

Curcumin: No data

Vitamin D reduces expression of the CCL8 gene

Effects of vitamin D supplementation on alveolar macrophage gene expression: preliminary results of a randomized, controlled trial[109]

Gaba: no data found

15. CCL17 (CC chemokine ligand 17, TARC ABCD-2)

"This antimicrobial gene is one of several Cys-Cys (CC) cytokine genes clustered on the q arm of chromosome 16. Cytokines are a family of secreted proteins involved in immunoregulatory and inflammatory processes. The CC cytokines are proteins characterized by two adjacent cysteines. The cytokine encoded by this gene displays chemotactic activity for T lymphocytes, but not monocytes or granulocytes. The product of this gene binds to chemokine receptors CCR4 and CCR8." (*CCL17, National Institutes of Health*)

CCL17 predicts mild to severe Covid-19

Serum CCL17 level becomes a predictive marker to distinguish between mild/moderate and severe/critical disease in patients with COVID-19[110]

Glucose: no data found

Cannabinoids down-regulate CCL17

Polyphenols and Cannabidiol Modulate Transcriptional Regulation of Th1/Th2 Inflammatory Genes Related to Canine Atopic Dermatitis[111]

Curcumin reduces production of CCL17

IL-17 stimulates the expression of CCL2 in cardiac myocytes via Act1/TRAF6/p38MAPK-dependent AP-1 activation[112]

Low Vitamin D raise CCL17 (TARC) Levels

107 Varol C, Zvibel I, Spektor L, Mantelmacher FD, Vugman M, Thurm T, Khatib M, Elmaliah E, Halpern Z, Fishman S. Long-acting glucose-dependent insulinotropic polypeptide ameliorates obesity-induced adipose tissue inflammation. J Immunol. 2014 Oct 15;193(8):4002-9. doi: 10.4049/jimmunol.1401149. Epub 2014 Sep 12. PMID: 25217161.

108 Gaffal E, Cron M, Glodde N, Tüting T. Anti-inflammatory activity of topical THC in DNFB-mediated mouse allergic contact dermatitis independent of CB1 and CB2 receptors. Allergy. 2013 Aug;68(8):994-1000. doi: 10.1111/all.12183. Epub 2013 Jul 29. PMID: 23889474.

109 Gerke AK, Pezzulo AA, Tang F, Cavanaugh JE, Bair TB, Phillips E, Powers LS, Monick MM. Effects of vitamin D supplementation on alveolar macrophage gene expression: preliminary results of a randomized, controlled trial. Multidiscip Respir Med. 2014 Mar 26;9(1):18. doi: 10.1186/2049-6958-9-18. PMID: 24669961; PMCID: PMC3986866.

110 Sugiyama M, Kinoshita N, Ide S, Nomoto H, Nakamoto T, Saito S, Ishikane M, Kutsuna S, Hayakawa K, Hashimoto M, Suzuki M, Izumi S, Hojo M, Tsuchiya K, Gatanaga H, Takasaki J, Usami M, Kano T, Yanai H, Nishida N, Kanto T, Sugiyama H, Ohmagari N, Mizokami M. Serum CCL17 level becomes a predictive marker to distinguish between mild/moderate and severe/critical disease in patients with COVID-19. Gene. 2021 Jan 15;766:145145. doi: 10.1016/j.gene.2020.145145. Epub 2020 Sep 14. PMID: 32941953; PMCID: PMC7489253.

111 Massimini M, Dalle Vedove E, Bachetti B, Di Pierro F, Ribecco C, D'Addario C, Pucci M. Polyphenols and Cannabidiol Modulate Transcriptional Regulation of Th1/Th2 Inflammatory Genes Related to Canine Atopic Dermatitis. Front Vet Sci. 2021 Mar 5;8:606197. doi: 10.3389/fvets.2021.606197. PMID: 33763461; PMCID: PMC7982812.

112 Xiao Huang, Zhuolun Li, Xinhe Shen, Na Nie, Yan Shen, IL-17 upregulates MCP-1 expression via Act1 / TRAF6 / TAK1 in experimental autoimmune myocarditis, Cytokine, 10.1016/j.cyto.2022.155823, 152, (155823), (2022). Crossref

Infantile atopic dermatitis: Serum vitamin D, zinc and TARC levels and their relationship with disease phenotype and severity[113]
Gaba: no data found

16. CCL20 (MIP-3a)

"CCL20 is expressed in thymus, in lymph nodes, and at high levels in epithelium associated with MALT. Inflammatory cytokines and lipopolysaccharide (LPS) induce the expression of CCL20 by peripheral blood mononuclear cells (PBMCs), endothelial and epithelial cells, monocyte and macrophage cell lines, and neutrophils"[114]

Covid-19 increases CCL20 expression
COVID-19 severity correlates with airway epithelium–immune cell interactions identified by single-cell analysis[115]

High Glucose induces CCL20
High Glucose Induces CCL20 in Proximal Tubular Cells via Activation of the KCa3.1 Channel[116]

Cannabinoids: no data found
Curcumin: no data found

Vitamin D down-regulates CCL20
Vitamin D down-regulates the expression of some Th17 cell-related cytokines, key inflammatory chemokines, and chemokine receptors in experimental autoimmune encephalomyelitis[117]
Gaba: no data found

17. CCL24 [myeloid progenitor inhibitory factor 2 (MPIF-2) or eosinophil chemotactic protein 2 (eotaxin-2)]

"Enables cytokine activity. Involved in positive regulation of angiogenesis and positive regulation of inflammatory response. Acts upstream of or within chemotaxis and positive regulation of eosinophil migration. Predicted to be located in extracellular region. Predicted to be active in extracellular space. Human ortholog(s) of this gene implicated in asthma and rhinitis." (*CCL24, National Library of Medicine, NIH*)

"CCL24 plays an important role in pathological processes of skin and lung inflammation and fibrosis. Inhibition of CCL24 by CM-101 mAb can be potentially beneficial for therapeutic use in SSc patients." (*Blockade of CCL24 with a monoclonal antibody ameliorates experimental dermal and pulmonary fibrosis*)

CCL24 mediates Covid-19 inflammation and severity
Early Th2 inflammation in the upper respiratory mucosa as a predictor of severe COVID-19 and modulation by early treatment with inhaled corticosteroids: a mechanistic analysis[118]

113 Esenboga S, Cetinkaya PG, Sahiner N, Birben E, Soyer O, Sekerel BE, Sahiner UM. Infantile atopic dermatitis: Serum vitamin D, zinc and TARC levels and their relationship with disease phenotype and severity. Allergol Immunopathol (Madr). 2021 May 1;49(3):162-168. doi: 10.15586/aei.v49i3.191. PMID: 33938202.

114 Ronald L. Rabin, in Encyclopedia of Hormones, 2003

115 Chua, R.L., Lukassen, S., Trump, S. et al. COVID-19 severity correlates with airway epithelium–immune cell interactions identified by single-cell analysis. Nat Biotechnol 38, 970–979 (2020). https://doi.org/10.1038/s41587-020-0602-4

116 Huang, Chunling et al. "High glucose induces CCL20 in proximal tubular cells via activation of the KCa3.1 channel." PloS one vol. 9,4 e95173. 14 Apr. 2014, doi:10.1371/journal.pone.0095173

117 Jafarzadeh A, Azizi SV, Arabi Z, Ahangar-Parvin R, Mohammadi-Kordkhayli M, Larussa T, Khatami F, Nemati M. Vitamin D down-regulates the expression of some Th17 cell-related cytokines, key inflammatory chemokines, and chemokine receptors in experimental autoimmune encephalomyelitis. Nutr Neurosci. 2019 Oct;22(10):725-737. doi: 10.1080/1028415X.2018.1436237. Epub 2018 Feb 15. PMID: 29447086.

118 Baker JR, Mahdi M, Nicolau DV Jr, Ramakrishnan S, Barnes PJ, Simpson JL, Cass SP, Russell REK, Donnelly LE, Bafadhel M. Early Th2 inflammation in the upper respiratory mucosa as a predictor of severe COVID-19 and modulation by early treatment with inhaled corticosteroids: a mechanistic analysis. Lancet Respir Med. 2022 Jun;10(6):545-556. doi:

High Glucose increases CCL24
CCL24 Protects Renal Function by Controlling Inflammation in Podocytes[119]
Cannabinoid receptor CB2 controls MPIF-2
The CB2 Cannabinoid Receptor Controls Myeloid Progenitor Trafficking[120]
Curcumin: no data found
Vitamin D: no data found
Gaba: no data found

18. CXCL1 [(C-X-C motif) ligand 1]

"This antimicrobial gene encodes a member of the CXC subfamily of chemokines. The encoded protein is a secreted growth factor that signals through the G-protein coupled receptor, CXC receptor 2. This protein plays a role in inflammation and as a chemoattractant for neutrophils. Aberrant expression of this protein is associated with the growth and progression of certain tumors. A naturally occurring processed form of this protein has increased chemotactic activity." *(CXCL1, National Library of Medicine, NIH)*

CXCL1 is expressed in Covid-19
COVID-19 severity correlates with airway epithelium-immune cell interactions identified by single-cell analysis[121]
High Glucose and obesity linked to increased CXCL1 expression
Increased serum CXCL1 and CXCL5 are linked to obesity, hyperglycemia, and impaired islet function[122]
Cannabinoids suppresses CXCL1
Critical Role of Mast Cells and Peroxisome Proliferator-Activated Receptor γ in the Induction of Myeloid-Derived Suppressor Cells by Marijuana Cannabidiol In Vivo[123]
Curcumin down-regulates CXCL1
Curcumin downregulates the inflammatory cytokines CXCL1 and -2 in breast cancer cells via NFκB[124]

Vitamin D upregulates CXCL1

10.1016/S2213-2600(22)00002-9. Epub 2022 Apr 7. Erratum in: Lancet Respir Med. 2022 Jun;10(6):e60. PMID: 35397798; PMCID: PMC8989397.

119 Wang Y, Wu X, Geng M, Ding J, Lv K, Du H, Ding J, Pei W, Hu X, Gu J, Wang L, Zhang Y, Gao J. CCL24 Protects Renal Function by Controlling Inflammation in Podocytes. Dis Markers. 2021 Jun 16;2021:8837825. doi: 10.1155/2021/8837825. PMID: 34221188; PMCID: PMC8221868.

120 Palazuelos J, Davoust N, Julien B, Hatterer E, Aguado T, Mechoulam R, Benito C, Romero J, Silva A, Guzmán M, Nataf S, Galve-Roperh I. The CB(2) cannabinoid receptor controls myeloid progenitor trafficking: involvement in the pathogenesis of an animal model of multiple sclerosis. J Biol Chem. 2008 May 9;283(19):13320-9. doi: 10.1074/jbc.M707960200. Epub 2008 Mar 11. PMID: 18334483.

121 Chua RL, Lukassen S, Trump S, Hennig BP, Wendisch D, Pott F, Debnath O, Thürmann L, Kurth F, Völker MT, Kazmierski J, Timmermann B, Twardziok S, Schneider S, Machleidt F, Müller-Redetzky H, Maier M, Krannich A, Schmidt S, Balzer F, Liebig J, Loske J, Suttorp N, Eils J, Ishaque N, Liebert UG, von Kalle C, Hocke A, Witzenrath M, Goffinet C, Drosten C, Laudi S, Lehmann I, Conrad C, Sander LE, Eils R. COVID-19 severity correlates with airway epithelium-immune cell interactions identified by single-cell analysis. Nat Biotechnol. 2020 Aug;38(8):970-979. doi: 10.1038/s41587-020-0602-4. Epub 2020 Jun 26. PMID: 32591762.

122 Nunemaker CS, Chung HG, Verrilli GM, Corbin KL, Upadhye A, Sharma PR. Increased serum CXCL1 and CXCL5 are linked to obesity, hyperglycemia, and impaired islet function. J Endocrinol. 2014 Aug;222(2):267-76. doi: 10.1530/JOE-14-0126. Epub 2014 Jun 13. PMID: 24928936; PMCID: PMC4135511.

123 Hegde VL, Singh UP, Nagarkatti PS, Nagarkatti M. Critical Role of Mast Cells and Peroxisome Proliferator-Activated Receptor γ in the Induction of Myeloid-Derived Suppressor Cells by Marijuana Cannabidiol In Vivo. J Immunol. 2015 Jun 1;194(11):5211-22. doi: 10.4049/jimmunol.1401844. Epub 2015 Apr 27. PMID: 25917103; PMCID: PMC4433789.

124 Beatrice E. Bachmeier, Isabelle V. Mohrenz, Valentina Mirisola, Erwin Schleicher, Francesco Romeo, Clara Höhneke, Marianne Jochum, Andreas G. Nerlich, Ulrich Pfeffer, Curcumin downregulates the inflammatory cytokines CXCL1 and -2 in breast cancer cells via NFκB, Carcinogenesis, Volume 29, Issue 4, April 2008, Pages 779–789, https://doi.org/10.1093/carcin/bgm248

Primary 1,25-dihydroxyvitamin D3 response of the interleukin 8 gene cluster in human monocyte- and macrophage-like cells[125]

Gaba reduces CXCL1

Immunomodulatory Properties of a γ-Aminobutyric Acid-Enriched Strawberry Juice Produced by Levilactobacillus brevis CRL 2013[126]

19. CXCL2 (Chemokine (C-X-C motif) ligand 2 , macrophage inflammatory protein 2-alpha (MIP2-alpha), Growth-regulated protein beta (Gro-beta) and Gro oncogene-2 (Gro-2)
"Neutrophils and the CXC2-CXCR2 axis. Both CXCL1 and CXCL2 act through CXCR2 expressed on neutrophils. Antibody neutralization of CXCR2 has confirmed the need for neutrophil recruitment in models of P. aeruginosa (Tsai et al., 2000). Consistent with this, CXCR2 deficient mice have severely perturbed recruitment of neutrophils (and exudate macrophages) resulting in bacterial outgrowth in pneumococcal pneumonia (Herbold et al., 2010)." *(CXCL2 - an overview ScienceDirect Topics)*

Covid-19 raises CXCL2

Chemokines and chemokine receptors during COVID-19 infection[127]

CXCL2 is up-regulated in obesity

Roles of Chemokine Ligand-2 (CXCL2) and Neutrophils in Influencing Endothelial Cell Function and Inflammation of Human Adipose Tissue[128]

Cannabinoid receptor CB2 inhibits CXCL2

Activation of cannabinoid 2 receptors protects against cerebral ischemia by inhibiting neutrophil recruitment[129]

Curcumin inhibits CXCL2

Curcumin Inhibits 5-Fluorouracil-induced Up-regulation of CXCL1 and CXCL2 of the Colon Associated with Attenuation of Diarrhoea Development[130]

Vitamin D inhibits CXCL2

Vitamin D3-vitamin D receptor axis suppresses pulmonary emphysema by maintaining alveolar macrophage homeostasis and function[131]

Gaba interferes with the production of CXCL2

125 Ryynänen J, Carlberg C. Primary 1,25-dihydroxyvitamin D3 response of the interleukin 8 gene cluster in human monocyte- and macrophage-like cells. PLoS One. 2013 Oct 21;8(10):e78170. doi: 10.1371/journal.pone.0078170. PMID: 24250750; PMCID: PMC3824026.

126 Cataldo PG, Villena J, Elean M, Savoy de Giori G, Saavedra L, Hebert EM. Immunomodulatory Properties of a γ-Aminobutyric Acid-Enriched Strawberry Juice Produced by Levilactobacillus brevis CRL 2013. Front Microbiol. 2020 Dec 17;11:610016. doi: 10.3389/fmicb.2020.610016. PMID: 33391235; PMCID: PMC7773669.

127 Khalil BA, Elemam NM, Maghazachi AA. Chemokines and chemokine receptors during COVID-19 infection. Comput Struct Biotechnol J. 2021;19:976-988. doi: 10.1016/j.csbj.2021.01.034. Epub 2021 Jan 27. PMID: 33558827; PMCID: PMC7859556.

128 Christine Rouault, Vanessa Pellegrinelli, Raphaela Schilch, Aurélie Cotillard, Christine Poitou, Joan Tordjman, Henrike Sell, Karine Clément, Danièle Lacasa, Roles of Chemokine Ligand-2 (CXCL2) and Neutrophils in Influencing Endothelial Cell Function and Inflammation of Human Adipose Tissue, Endocrinology, Volume 154, Issue 3, 1 March 2013, Pages 1069–1079, https://doi.org/10.1210/en.2012-1415

129 Murikinati S, Jüttler E, Keinert T, Ridder DA, Muhammad S, Waibler Z, Ledent C, Zimmer A, Kalinke U, Schwaninger M. Activation of cannabinoid 2 receptors protects against cerebral ischemia by inhibiting neutrophil recruitment. FASEB J. 2010 Mar;24(3):788-98. doi: 10.1096/fj.09-141275. Epub 2009 Nov 2. PMID: 19884325.

130 Sakai H, Kai Y, Oguchi A, Kimura M, Tabata S, Yaegashi M, Saito T, Sato K, Sato F, Yumoto T, Narita M. Curcumin Inhibits 5-Fluorouracil-induced Up-regulation of CXCL1 and CXCL2 of the Colon Associated with Attenuation of Diarrhoea Development. Basic Clin Pharmacol Toxicol. 2016 Dec;119(6):540-547. doi: 10.1111/bcpt.12619. Epub 2016 Jul 26. PMID: 27194111.

131 Hu G, Dong T, Wang S, Jing H, Chen J. Vitamin D3-vitamin D receptor axis suppresses pulmonary emphysema by maintaining alveolar macrophage homeostasis and function. EBioMedicine. 2019 Jul;45:563-577. doi: 10.1016/j.ebiom.2019.06.039. Epub 2019 Jul 2. PMID: 31278070; PMCID: PMC6642288.

**Anti-inflammatory effects of the GABA(B) receptor agonist baclofen in allergic contact dermatitis**[132]

20. CXCL8 (C-X-C motif chemokine ligand 8; Interleukin 8)

"The protein encoded by this gene is a member of the CXC chemokine family and is a major mediator of the inflammatory response. The encoded protein is commonly referred to as interleukin-8 (IL-8). IL-8 is secreted by mononuclear macrophages, neutrophils, eosinophils, T lymphocytes, epithelial cells, and fibroblasts. It functions as a chemotactic factor by guiding the neutrophils to the site of infection. Bacterial and viral products rapidly induce IL-8 expression. IL-8 also participates with other cytokines in the proinflammatory signaling cascade and plays a role in systemic inflammatory response syndrome (SIRS). This gene is believed to play a role in the pathogenesis of the lower respiratory tract infection bronchiolitis, a common respiratory tract disease caused by the respiratory syncytial virus (RSV). The overproduction of this proinflammatory protein is thought to cause the lung inflammation associated with csytic fibrosis. This proinflammatory protein is also suspected of playing a role in coronary artery disease and endothelial dysfunction." _**(CXCL8, National Library of Medicine, NIH)**_

Covid-19 raises CXCL8

**The cytokine storm in COVID-19: An overview of the involvement of the chemokine/chemokine-receptor system**[133]

High Glucose induces CXCL8

**Insulin induces monocytic CXCL8 secretion by the mitogenic signalling pathway**[134]

Cannabinoids reduce CXCL8 (interleukin-8), but increase in higher doses

**Effects of cannabidiol on activated immune-inflammatory pathways in major depressivepatients and healthy controls**[135]

Curcumin inhibits CXCL8 (interleukin 8)

**Rationale and Means to Target Pro-Inflammatory Interleukin-8 (CXCL8) Signaling in Cancer**[136]

Vitamin D down-regulates CXCL8 (interleukin 8)

**Down-regulation of IL-8 by high-dose vitamin D is specific to hyperinflammatory macrophages and involves mechanisms beyond up-regulation of DUSP1**[137]

Gaba signaling might play a key role in CXCL8 (interleukin 8)

**Serum Levels and in vitro CX3CL1 (Fractalkine), CXCL8, and IL-10 Synthesis in Phytohemaglutinin-Stimulated and Non-stimulated Peripheral Blood Mononuclear Cells in Subjects With Schizophrenia**[138]

132 Duthey B, Hübner A, Diehl S, Boehncke S, Pfeffer J, Boehncke WH. Anti-inflammatory effects of the GABA(B) receptor agonist baclofen in allergic contact dermatitis. Exp Dermatol. 2010 Jul 1;19(7):661-6. doi: 10.1111/j.1600-0625.2010.01076.x. Epub 2010 Feb 25. PMID: 20201957.

133 Coperchini F, Chiovato L, Croce L, Magri F, Rotondi M. The cytokine storm in COVID-19: An overview of the involvement of the chemokine/chemokine-receptor system. Cytokine Growth Factor Rev. 2020 Jun;53:25-32. doi: 10.1016/j.cytogfr.2020.05.003. Epub 2020 May 11. PMID: 32446778; PMCID: PMC7211650.

134 Wurm S, Neumeier M, Weigert J, Wanninger J, Gerl M, Gindner A, Schäffler A, Aslanidis C, Schölmerich J, Buechler C. Insulin induces monocytic CXCL8 secretion by the mitogenic signalling pathway. Cytokine. 2008 Oct;44(1):185-90. doi: 10.1016/j.cyto.2008.08.003. Epub 2008 Sep 11. PMID: 18789871.

135 Rachayon M, Jirakran K, Sodsai P, Klinchanhom S, Sughondhabirom A, Plaimas K, Suratanee A, Maes M. In Vitro Effects of Cannabidiol on Activated Immune-Inflammatory Pathways in Major Depressive Patients and Healthy Controls. Pharmaceuticals (Basel). 2022 Mar 26;15(4):405. doi: 10.3390/ph15040405. PMID: 35455402; PMCID: PMC9032852.

136 Campbell LM, Maxwell PJ, Waugh DJ. Rationale and Means to Target Pro-Inflammatory Interleukin-8 (CXCL8) Signaling in Cancer. Pharmaceuticals (Basel). 2013 Aug 6;6(8):929-59. doi: 10.3390/ph6080929. PMID: 24276377; PMCID: PMC3817732.

137 Dauletbaev N, Herscovitch K, Das M, Chen H, Bernier J, Matouk E, Bérubé J, Rousseau S, Lands LC. Down-regulation of IL-8 by high-dose vitamin D is specific to hyperinflammatory macrophages and involves mechanisms beyond up-regulation of DUSP1. Br J Pharmacol. 2015 Oct;172(19):4757-71. doi: 10.1111/bph.13249. PMID: 26178144; PMCID: PMC4594277.

138 Arabska J, Wysokiński A, Brzezińska-Błaszczyk E, Kozłowska E. Serum Levels and in vitro CX3CL1 (Fractalkine), CXCL8, and IL-10 Synthesis in Phytohemaglutinin-Stimulated and Non-stimulated Peripheral Blood Mononuclear Cells in Subjects With Schizophrenia. Front Psychiatry. 2022 Jun 17;13:845136. doi: 10.3389/fpsyt.2022.845136. PMID: 35782435;

21. CXCL9 (C-X-C motif chemokine ligand 9)

"This antimicrobial gene is part of a chemokine superfamily that encodes secreted proteins involved in immunoregulatory and inflammatory processes. The protein encoded is thought to be involved in T cell trafficking. The encoded protein binds to C-X-C motif chemokine 3 and is a chemoattractant for lymphocytes but not for neutrophils." (CXCL9. National Library of Medicine, NIH)

Covid-19 up-regulates CXCL9

The Pro-Inflammatory Chemokines CXCL9, CXCL10 and CXCL11 Are Upregulated Following SARS-CoV-2 Infection in an AKT-Dependent Manner[139]

High Glucose increases CXCL9

Glucose metabolism controls disease-specific signatures of macrophage effector functions[140]

Cannabinoids inhibit CXCL9.

Efficacy of cannabidiol treatment in experimental MS is due to immunosuppressive activity of myeloid cells in CNS downregulating recruitment of CD4+ T cells, proinflammatory chemokines and gasdermin D expression[141]

Curcumin inhibits CXCL9

Curcumin inhibits interferon-γ signaling in colonic epithelial cells[142]

Vitamin D decreases CXCL9

Vitamin D accelerates resolution of inflammatory responses during tuberculosis treatment[143]

Gaba receptor antagonist reduces CXCL9

Anti-inflammatory effects of the GABA(B) receptor agonist baclofen in allergic contact dermatitis[144]

22. CXCL10 (C-X-C motif chemokine ligand 10, Interferon gamma-induced protein 10 (IP-10) or small-inducible cytokine B10)

"This antimicrobial gene encodes a chemokine of the CXC subfamily and ligand for the receptor CXCR3. Binding of this protein to CXCR3 results in pleiotropic effects, including stimulation of monocytes, natural killer and T-cell migration, and modulation of adhesion molecule expression. This gene may also be a key regulator of the 'cytokine storm' immune response to SARS-CoV-2 infection." (CXCL10. *National Library of Medicine, NIH*)

Covid-19 raises CXCL10 (IP-10)

PMCID: PMC9247257.

139 Callahan V, Hawks S, Crawford MA, Lehman CW, Morrison HA, Ivester HM, Akhrymuk I, Boghdeh N, Flor R, Finkielstein CV, Allen IC, Weger-Lucarelli J, Duggal N, Hughes MA, Kehn-Hall K. The Pro-Inflammatory Chemokines CXCL9, CXCL10 and CXCL11 Are Upregulated Following SARS-CoV-2 Infection in an AKT-Dependent Manner. Viruses. 2021 Jun 3;13(6):1062. doi: 10.3390/v13061062. PMID: 34205098; PMCID: PMC8226769.

140 Watanabe R, Hilhorst M, Zhang H, Zeisbrich M, Berry GJ, Wallis BB, Harrison DG, Giacomini JC, Goronzy JJ, Weyand CM. Glucose metabolism controls disease-specific signatures of macrophage effector functions. JCI Insight. 2018 Oct 18;3(20):e123047. doi: 10.1172/jci.insight.123047. PMID: 30333306; PMCID: PMC6237479.

141 Efficacy of cannabidiol treatment in experimental MS is due to immunosuppressive activity of myeloid cells in CNS downregulating recruitment of CD4+ T cells, proinflammatory chemokines and gasdermin D expression Nicholas Dopkins, Kiesha Wilson, Kathryn Miranda, Prakash S Nagarkatti, Mitzi Nagarkatti The Journal of Immunology May 1, 2020, 204 (1 Supplement) 142.26;

142 Midura-Kiela MT, Radhakrishnan VM, Larmonier CB, Laubitz D, Ghishan FK, Kiela PR. Curcumin inhibits interferon-γ signaling in colonic epithelial cells. Am J Physiol Gastrointest Liver Physiol. 2012 Jan 1;302(1):G85-96. doi: 10.1152/ajpgi.00275.2011. Epub 2011 Oct 28. PMID: 22038826; PMCID: PMC3345961.

143 Coussens AK, Wilkinson RJ, Hanifa Y, Nikolayevskyy V, Elkington PT, Islam K, Timms PM, Venton TR, Bothamley GH, Packe GE, Darmalingam M, Davidson RN, Milburn HJ, Baker LV, Barker RD, Mein CA, Bhaw-Rosun L, Nuamah R, Young DB, Drobniewski FA, Griffiths CJ, Martineau AR. Vitamin D accelerates resolution of inflammatory responses during tuberculosis treatment. Proc Natl Acad Sci U S A. 2012 Sep 18;109(38):15449-54. doi: 10.1073/pnas.1200072109. Epub 2012 Sep 4. PMID: 22949664; PMCID: PMC3458393.

144 Duthey B, Hübner A, Diehl S, Boehncke S, Pfeffer J, Boehncke WH. Anti-inflammatory effects of the GABA(B) receptor agonist baclofen in allergic contact dermatitis. Exp Dermatol. 2010 Jul 1;19(7):661-6. doi: 10.1111/j.1600-0625.2010.01076.x. Epub 2010 Feb 25. PMID: 20201957.

Observational cohort study of IP-10's potential as a biomarker to aid in inflammation regulation within a clinical decision support protocol for patients with severe COVID-19[145]

Glucose increases secretion of CXCL10 (IP-10)

Increased secretion of IP-10 from monocytes under hyperglycemia is via the TLR2 and TLR4 pathway[146]

Cannabinoids decrease CXCL10 (IP-10)

Δ9-Tetrahydrocannabinol (THC) Impairs CD8+ T Cell-Mediated Activation of Astrocytes[147]

Curcumin reduces CXCL10 (IP-10)

The anti-inflammatory activity of curcumin protects the genital mucosal epithelial barrier from disruption and blocks replication of HIV-1 and HSV-2[148]

Vitamin D deficiency increases CXCL10 (IP-10)

Correction of vitamin D deficiency facilitated suppression of IP-10 and DPP IV levels in patients with chronic hepatitis C: A randomised double-blinded, placebo-control trial[149]

Gaba decreases CXCL10 (IP-10)

Anti-inflammatory effects of the GABA(B) receptor agonist baclofen in allergic contact dermatitis[150]

23. CSF2/GM-CSF (colony-stimulating factor 2 or Granulocyte-macrophage colony-stimulating factor)

"GM-CSF was originally identified as a colony stimulating factor (CSF) because of its ability to induce granulocyte and macrophage populations from precursor cells. Multiple studies have demonstrated that GM-CSF is also an immune-modulatory cytokine, capable of affecting not only the phenotype of myeloid lineage cells, but also T-cell activation through various myeloid intermediaries. This property has been implicated in the sustenance of several autoimmune diseases like arthritis and multiple sclerosis. In contrast, several studies using animal models have shown that GM-CSF is also capable of suppressing many autoimmune diseases such as Crohn's disease, Type-1 diabetes, Myasthenia gravis and experimental autoimmune thyroiditis. Knockout mouse studies have suggested that the role of GM-CSF in maintaining granulocyte and macrophage populations in the physiological steady state is largely redundant. Instead, its immune-modulatory role plays a significant role in the development or resolution of autoimmune diseases." (*GM-CSF: An immune modulatory cytokine that can suppress autoimmunity*[151])

Covid-19 can raise CSF2 (GM-CSF) high enough to cause damage

---

145 Shaul Lev, Tamar Gottesman, Gal Sahaf Levin, Doron Lederfein, Evgeny Berkov, Dror Diker, Aliza Zaidman, Amir Nutman, Tahel Ilan Ber, Alon Angel, Lior Kellerman, Eran Barash, Roy Navon, Boaz Tadmor. Published: January 12, 2021. https://doi.org/10.1371/journal.pone.0245296

146 Sridevi Devaraj, Ishwarlal Jialal,Increased secretion of IP-10 from monocytes under hyperglycemia is via the TLR2 and TLR4 pathway, Cytokine, Volume 47, Issue 1, 2009,Pages 6-10,ISSN 1043-4666,https://doi.org/10.1016/j.cyto.2009.02.004.

147 Henriquez JE, Bach AP, Matos-Fernandez KM, Crawford RB, Kaminski NE. Δ9-Tetrahydrocannabinol (THC) Impairs CD8+ T Cell-Mediated Activation of Astrocytes. J Neuroimmune Pharmacol. 2020 Dec;15(4):863-874. doi: 10.1007/s11481-020-09912-z. Epub 2020 Mar 26. PMID: 32215844; PMCID: PMC7529688.

148 Ferreira VH, Nazli A, Dizzell SE, Mueller K, Kaushic C. The anti-inflammatory activity of curcumin protects the genital mucosal epithelial barrier from disruption and blocks replication of HIV-1 and HSV-2. PLoS One. 2015 Apr 9;10(4):e0124903. doi: 10.1371/journal.pone.0124903. PMID: 25856395; PMCID: PMC4391950.

149 Komolmit, Piyawat et al. "Correction of vitamin D deficiency facilitated suppression of IP-10 and DPP IV levels in patients with chronic hepatitis C: A randomised double-blinded, placebo-control trial." PloS one vol. 12,4 e0174608. 4 Apr. 2017, doi:10.1371/journal.pone.0174608

150 Duthey B, Hübner A, Diehl S, Boehncke S, Pfeffer J, Boehncke WH. Anti-inflammatory effects of the GABA(B) receptor agonist baclofen in allergic contact dermatitis. Exp Dermatol. 2010 Jul 1;19(7):661-6. doi: 10.1111/j.1600-0625.2010.01076.x. Epub 2010 Feb 25. PMID: 20201957.

151 Bhattacharya P, Thiruppathi M, Elshabrawy HA, Alharshawi K, Kumar P, Prabhakar BS. GM-CSF: An immune modulatory cytokine that can suppress autoimmunity. Cytokine. 2015 Oct;75(2):261-71. doi: 10.1016/j.cyto.2015.05.030. Epub 2015 Jun 22. PMID: 26113402; PMCID: PMC4553090.

Stimulating severe COVID-19: the potential role of GM-CSF[152]

Glucose raises CSF2 (GM-CSF) levels

Increased Levels of Serum Granulocyte-Macrophage Colony-Stimulating Factor Is Associated with Activated Peripheral Dendritic Cells in Type 2 Diabetes Subjects (CURES-99)[153]

Cannabinoids lower CSF2 (GM-CSF)

Oral administration of cannabis with lipids leads to high levels of cannabinoids in the intestinal lymphatic system and prominent immunomodulation[154]

Curcumin suppresses CSF2 (GM-CSF)

Curcumin inhibits the growth of liver cancer by impairing myeloid-derived suppressor cells in murine tumor tissues[155]

Vitamin D lowers levels of CSF2 (GM-CSF)

Vitamin d and serum cytokines in a randomized clinical trial[156]

Elevated CSF2 (GM-CSF) levels reduce Gaba

GM-CSF affects hypothalamic neurotransmitter levels in mice: involvement of interleukin-1[157]

24. Interleukin-1

"Interleukin-1 (IL-1) is the prototypic pro-inflammatory cytokine. There are two forms of IL-1, IL-1alpha and IL-1beta and in most studies, their biological activities are indistinguishable. IL-1 affects nearly every cell type, often in concert with another pro-inflammatory cytokine, tumor necrosis factor (TNF). Although IL-1 can upregulate host defenses and function as an immunoadjuvant, IL-1 is a highly inflammatory cytokine. The margin between clinical benefit and unacceptable toxicity in humans is exceedingly narrow. In contrast, agents that reduce the production and/or activity of IL-1 are likely to have an impact on clinical medicine. The synthesis, processing, secretion and activity of IL-1, particularly IL-1beta, are tightly regulated events. A unique aspect of cytokine biology is the naturally occurring IL-1 receptor antagonist (IL-1Ra). IL-1Ra is structurally similar to IL-1beta but lacking agonist activity is used in clinical trials to reduce disease severity." (*Interleukin 1, National Library of Medicine, NIH*)

Covid-19 raises interleukin-1

SARS-CoV-2 infection: The role of cytokines in COVID-19 disease[158]

Interleukin-1 and interleukin 6 are triggers of the deadly COVID "cytokine storm:"

Impact of rare and common genetic variation in the interleukin-1 pathway on human cytokine responses[159]

High Glucose raises interleukin-1

152 Leavis HL, van de Veerdonk FL, Murthy S. Stimulating severe COVID-19: the potential role of GM-CSF antagonism. Lancet Respir Med. 2022 Mar;10(3):223-224. doi: 10.1016/S2213-2600(21)00539-7. Epub 2021 Dec 1. PMID: 34863335; PMCID: PMC8635456.

153 Surendar J, Mohan V, Pavankumar N, Babu S, Aravindhan V. Increased levels of serum granulocyte-macrophage colony-stimulating factor is associated with activated peripheral dendritic cells in type 2 diabetes subjects (CURES-99). Diabetes Technol Ther. 2012 Apr;14(4):344-9. doi: 10.1089/dia.2011.0182. Epub 2011 Dec 9. PMID: 22149626.

154 Zgair, A., Lee, J.B., Wong, J.C.M. et al. Oral administration of cannabis with lipids leads to high levels of cannabinoids in the intestinal lymphatic system and prominent immunomodulation. Sci Rep 7, 14542 (2017). https://doi.org/10.1038/s41598-017-15026-z

155 Tian S, Liao L, Zhou Q, Huang X, Zheng P, Guo Y, Deng T and Tian X: Curcumin inhibits the growth of liver cancer by impairing myeloid-derived suppressor cells in murine tumor tissues. Oncol Lett 21: 286, 2021

156 Yusupov E, Li-Ng M, Pollack S, Yeh JK, Mikhail M, Aloia JF. Vitamin d and serum cytokines in a randomized clinical trial. Int J Endocrinol. 2010;2010:305054. doi: 10.1155/2010/305054. Epub 2010 Aug 12. PMID: 20871847; PMCID: PMC2943086.

157 Bianchi M, Clavenna A, Bondiolotti GP, Ferrario P, Panerai AE. GM-CSF affects hypothalamic neurotransmitter levels in mice: involvement of interleukin-1. Neuroreport. 1997 Nov 10;8(16):3587-90. doi: 10.1097/00001756-199711100-00033. PMID: 9427331.

158 Costela-Ruiz, Víctor J et al. "SARS-CoV-2 infection: The role of cytokines in COVID-19 disease." Cytokine & growth factor reviews vol. 54 (2020): 62-75. doi:10.1016/j.cytogfr.2020.06.001

159 Van Deuren, R.C., Arts, P., Cavalli, G. et al. Impact of rare and common genetic variation in the interleukin-1 pathway on human cytokine responses. Genome Med 13, 94 (2021). https://doi.org/10.1186/s13073-021-00907-w

Glucose Induces IL-1α-Dependent Inflammation and Extracellular Matrix Proteins Expression and Deposition in Renal Tubular Epithial Cells in Diabetic Kidney Disease[160]

Cannabinoids lower interleukin-1

Cannabinoids as Key Regulators of Inflammasome Signaling: A Current Perspective

Immune Responses Regulated by Cannabidiol[161]

Curcumin blocks interleukin-1

Curcumin Blocks Interleukin-1 (IL-1) Signaling by Inhibiting the Recruitment of the IL-1 Receptor–Associated Kinase IRAK in Murine Thymoma EL-4 Cells[162]

Vitamin D inhibits interleukin-1

Vitamin D/VDR signaling inhibits LPS-induced IFNγ and IL-1β in Oral epithelia by regulating hypoxia-inducible factor-1α signaling pathway[163]

Interleukin-1 inhibits Gaba receptor

Interleukin-1beta inhibits gamma-aminobutyric acid type A (GABA(A)) receptor current in cultured hippocampal neurons[164]

25. Interleukin-2

"The existence of interleukin (IL)-2 has been recognized for over 25 years, and it remains one of the most extensively studied cytokines. Here we present a broad overview of IL-2 history, functional activities, biological sources, regulation and applications to disease treatment. IL-2 exerts a wide spectrum of effects on the immune system, and it plays crucial roles in regulating both immune activation and homeostasis." (***Overview of interleukin-2 function, production and clinical applications. National Library of Medicine, NIH***)

Covid-19 increases interleukin 2

How COVID-19 induces cytokine storm with high mortality[165]

Glucose elevates interleukin-2

Elevated adipose tissue assiated IL-2 expression in obesity correlates with metabolic inflammation and insulin resistance[166]

Cannabinoids reduce interleukin-2

Delta-9-tetrahydrocannabinol treatment results in a suppression of interleukin-2-induced cellular activities in human and murine lymphocytes[167]

The Profile of Immune Modulation by Cannabidiol (CBD) Involves Deregulation of Nuclear Factor of Activated T Cells (NFAT)[168]

---

160 Salti Talal, Khazim Khaled, Haddad Rami, Campisi-Pinto Salvatore, Bar-Sela Gil, Cohen Idan. Frontiers in Immunology. Volume 11, 2020

161 Nichols JM, and Kaplan BLF (2020) Immune responses regulated by cannabidiol, Cannabis and Cannabinoid Research 5:1, 12–31, DOI: 10.1089/can.2018.0073.

162 Jurrmann N, Brigelius-Flohé R, Böl GF. Curcumin blocks interleukin-1 (IL-1) signaling by inhibiting the recruitment of the IL-1 receptor-associated kinase IRAK in murine thymoma EL-4 cells. J Nutr. 2005 Aug;135(8):1859-64. doi: 10.1093/jn/135.8.1859. PMID: 16046709.

163 Ge, X., Wang, L., Li, M. et al. Vitamin D/VDR signaling inhibits LPS-induced IFNγ and IL-1β in Oral epithelia by regulating hypoxia-inducible factor-1α signaling pathway. Cell Commun Signal 17, 18 (2019). https://doi.org/10.1186/s12964-019-0331-9

164 Wang S, Cheng Q, Malik S, Yang J. Interleukin-1beta inhibits gamma-aminobutyric acid type A (GABA(A)) receptor current in cultured hippocampal neurons. J Pharmacol Exp Ther. 2000 Feb;292(2):497-504. PMID: 10640285.

165 Hojyo, S., Uchida, M., Tanaka, K. et al. How COVID-19 induces cytokine storm with high mortality. Inflamm Regener 40, 37 (2020). https://doi.org/10.1186/s41232-020-00146-3

166 Hojyo, S., Uchida, M., Tanaka, K. et al. How COVID-19 induces cytokine storm with high mortality. Inflamm Regener 40, 37 (2020). https://doi.org/10.1186/s41232-020-00146-3

167 Kirk Trisler, Steven Specter, International Journal of Immunopharmacology. Volume 16, Issue 7, 1994, Pages 593-603,ISSN 0192-0561, https://doi.org/10.1016/0192-0561(94)90110-4.

168 Kaplan BL, Springs AE, Kaminski NE. The profile of immune modulation by cannabidiol (CBD) involves deregulation of nuclear factor of activated T cells (NFAT). Biochem Pharmacol. 2008 Sep 15;76(6):726-37. doi: 10.1016/j.bcp.2008.06.022. Epub 2008 Jul 8. PMID: 18656454; PMCID: PMC2748879.

Curcumin lowers interleukin-2
Curcumin blocks interleukin (IL)-2 signaling in T-lymphocytes by inhibiting IL-2 synthesis, CD25 expression, and IL-2 receptor signaling[169]
Vitamin D lowers interleukin-2
Transcriptional repression of the interleukin-2 gene by vitamin D3: direct inhibition of NFATp/AP-1 complex formation by a nuclear hormone receptor[170]
Gaba: no data found

26. Interleukin-5

"Interleukin-5 (IL-5) is a growth factor and chemoattractant for eosinophils and is thought to play an essential role in allergic rhinitis, eosinophilic esophagitis and idiopathic hypereosinophilic syndrome" (*Science Direct, Interleukin-5*)
Covid-19 raises interleukin-5
Interleukin-5, Interleukin-6 and Eosinophils in COVID-19 Egyptian Patients: Potential Clues for Prognosis and Immunotherapy[171]
High Glucose increases interleukin-5
Proinflammatory cytokine polarization in type 2 diabetes[172]
Cannabinoids lower interleukin-5
Evaluation of Serum Cytokines Levels and the Role of Cannabidiol Treatment in Animal Model of Asthma[173]
Curcumin lowers interleukin-5
Curcumin suppresses ovalbumin-induced allergic conjunctivitis[174]
Vitamin D: inconclusive.
Different doses of supplemental vitamin D maintain interleukin-5 without altering skeletal muscle strength: a randomized, double-blind, placebo-controlled study in vitamin D sufficient adults[175]
Gaba: no data found

27. Interleukin-6

"COVID-19 has emerged as a global pandemic. It is mainly manifested as pneumonia which may deteriorate into severe respiratory failure. The major hallmark of the disease is the systemic inflammatory immune response characterized by Cytokine Storm (CS). CS is marked by elevated levels of inflammatory cytokines, mainly interleukin-6 (IL-6), IL-8, IL-10, tumour necrosis factor-α (TNF-α) and interferon-γ (IFN-γ). Of these, IL-6 is found to be significantly associated with higher mortality.

169 Forward NA, Conrad DM, Power Coombs MR, Doucette CD, Furlong SJ, Lin TJ, Hoskin DW. Curcumin blocks interleukin (IL)-2 signaling in T-lymphocytes by inhibiting IL-2 synthesis, CD25 expression, and IL-2 receptor signaling. Biochem Biophys Res Commun. 2011 Apr 22;407(4):801-6. doi: 10.1016/j.bbrc.2011.03.103. Epub 2011 Apr 2. PMID: 21443863.

170 ASM Journals. Molecular and Cellular Biology. Vol. 15, No. 10. 01 October 1995

171 International Journal of Medical Arts. Al-Azhar University (Damietta), Faculty of Medicine, Taha, Sara I.,El Sehsah, Eman M., Fouad, Shaimaa H., Ezzelregal, Hieba G., Moussa, Aya H., Abdalgeleel, Shaimaa A., Abdelmaksoud, Mariam F. 01/01/2022

172 Bahgat, Mervat M, and Dalia R Ibrahim. "Proinflammatory cytokine polarization in type 2 diabetes." Central-European journal of immunology vol. 45,2 (2020): 170-175. doi:10.5114/ceji.2020.97904

173 Vuolo, Francieli et al. "Evaluation of Serum Cytokines Levels and the Role of Cannabidiol Treatment in Animal Model of Asthma." Mediators of inflammation vol. 2015 (2015): 538670. doi:10.1155/2015/538670

174 Chung SH, Choi SH, Choi JA, Chuck RS, Joo CK. Curcumin suppresses ovalbumin-induced allergic conjunctivitis. Mol Vis. 2012;18:1966-72. Epub 2012 Jul 18. PMID: 22876123; PMCID: PMC3413438.

175 Barker T, Martins TB, Hill HR, Kjeldsberg CR, Henriksen VT, Dixon BM, Schneider ED, Dern A, Weaver LK. Different doses of supplemental vitamin D maintain interleukin-5 without altering skeletal muscle strength: a randomized, double-blind, placebo-controlled study in vitamin D sufficient adults. Nutr Metab (Lond). 2012 Mar 9;9(1):16. doi: 10.1186/1743-7075-9-16. PMID: 22405472; PMCID: PMC3325895.

IL-6 is also a robust marker for predicting disease prognosis and deterioration of clinical profile."
(Interleukin-6 Perpetrator of the COVID-19 Cytokine Storm)[176]

Covid-19 raises levels of interleukin-6
Interleukin-6 in Covid-19: A systematic review and meta-analysis[177]

High Glucose raises interleukin-6
Inflammatory Cytokine Concentrations Are Acutely Increased by Hyperglycemia in Humans[178]

Cannabinoids lower interleukin-6
Δ 9-Tetrahydrocannabinol Suppresses Monocyte-Mediated Astrocyte Production of Monocyte Chemoattractant Protein 1 and Interleukin-6 in a Toll-Like Receptor 7-Stimulated Human Coculture[179]

Cannabidiol selectively modulates interleukin (IL)-1β and IL-6 production in toll-like receptor activated human peripheral blood monocytes[180]

Curcumin inhibits interleukin-6
Curcumin: An Effective Inhibitor of Interleukin-6[181]

Vitamin D inhibits interleukin-6
Inhibitory effects of Vitamin D on inflammation and IL-6 release. A further support for COVID-19 management?[182]

Gaba inhibits interleukin-6
Gamma-aminobutyric acid inhibits synergistic interleukin-6 release but not transcriptional activation in astrocytoma cells[183]

28. IL-12 (interleukin-12)
"Interleukin-12 (IL-12) is a potent proinflammatory cytokine that enhances the cytotoxic activity of T lymphocytes and resting natural killer cells."[184]

Covid-19 raises interleukin-12 levels
Early Differences in Cytokine Production by Severity of Coronavirus Disease 2019[185]

High Glucose raises interleukin-12 levels
Elevated Glucose and Diabetes Promote Interleukin-12 Cytokine Gene Expression in Mouse Macrophages[186]

---

176 Shekhawat, Jyoti et al. "Interleukin-6 Perpetrator of the COVID-19 Cytokine Storm." Indian journal of clinical biochemistry : IJCB, vol. 36,4 1-11. 21 Jun. 2021, doi:10.1007/s12291-021-00989-8

177 Coomes EA, Haghbayan H. Interleukin-6 in Covid-19: A systematic review and meta-analysis. Rev Med Virol. 2020 Nov;30(6):1-9. doi: 10.1002/rmv.2141. Epub 2020 Aug 26. PMID: 32845568; PMCID: PMC7460877.

178 30 Sep 2002 https://doi.org/10.1161/01.CIR.0000034509.14906. AE Circulation. 2002;106:2067–2072

179 Rizzo MD, Crawford RB, Bach A, Sermet S, Amalfitano A, Kaminski NE. Δ9-Tetrahydrocannabinol Suppresses Monocyte-Mediated Astrocyte Production of Monocyte Chemoattractant Protein 1 and Interleukin-6 in a Toll-Like Receptor 7-Stimulated Human Coculture. J Pharmacol Exp Ther. 2019 Oct;371(1):191-201. doi: 10.1124/jpet.119.260661. Epub 2019 Aug 5. PMID: 31383729; PMCID: PMC7184191.

180 Sera Sermet, Jinpeng Li, Anthony Bach, Robert B. Crawford, Norbert E. Kaminski,Toxicology, Volume 464,2021,153016,ISSN 0300-483X, https://doi.org/10.1016/j.tox.2021.153016.

181 Ghandadi M, Sahebkar A. Curcumin: An Effective Inhibitor of Interleukin-6. Curr Pharm Des. 2017;23(6):921-931. doi: 10.2174/1381612822666161006151605. PMID: 27719643.

182 B. Orrù, J. Szekeres-Bartho, M. Bizzarri, A.M. Spiga, V. Unfer Eur Rev Med Pharmacol Sci. 2020. Vol. 24 - N. 15. Pages: 8187-8193. DOI: 10.26355/eurrev_202008_22507

183 Roach JD Jr, Aguinaldo GT, Jonnalagadda K, Hughes FM Jr, Spangelo BL. Gamma-aminobutyric acid inhibits synergistic interleukin-6 release but not transcriptional activation in astrocytoma cells. Neuroimmunomodulation. 2008;15(2):117-24. doi: 10.1159/000148194. Epub 2008 Aug 5. PMID: 18679050; PMCID: PMC2859952.

184 From: Pediatric Surgery (Seventh Edition), 2012

185 The Journal of Infectious Diseases, Volume 223, Issue 7, 1 April 2021, Pages 1145–1149, https://doi.org/10.1093/infdis/jiab005 Published: 07 January 2021

186 Yeshao Wen, Jiali Gu, Shu-Lian Li, Marpadga A. Reddy, Rama Natarajan, Jerry L. Nadler, Elevated Glucose and Diabetes Promote Interleukin-12 Cytokine Gene Expression in Mouse Macrophages, Endocrinology, Volume 147, Issue 5, 1 May 2006, Pages 2518–2525, https://doi.org/10.1210/en.2005-0519

Cannabinoids lower interleukin-12 levels
The Effect of Cannabis on the Clinical and Cytokine Profiles in Patients with Multiple Sclerosis[187]
Curcumin lowers interleukin-12 levels
Curcumin inhibits Th1 cytokine profile in CD4+ T cells by suppressing interleukin-12 production in macrophages[188]
Vitamin D lowers interleukin-12 levels
The Modulatory Effects of Vitamin D on the Expression of IL-12 and TGF-β in the Spinal Cord and Serum of Mice with Experimental Autoimmune Encephalomyelitis[189]
Gaba reduces interleukin-12 levels
GABA (A) receptor subunits RNA expression in mice peritoneal macrophages modulate their IL-6/IL-12 production[190]

29. IL-17, 17A (interleukin 17, 17a)

"IL-17 is a pro-inflammatory cytokine secreted by CD4 Th17 and CD8 Tc17 cells. Tumor growth is suppressed and MDSC levels are decreased in IL-17-deficient mice, while administration of IL-17 raises MDSC levels (He et al., 2010; Wang et al., 2009). Patients with gastrointestinal cancers show a strong positive correlation between serum IL-17 and MDSC levels, further supporting a role for IL-17 as an inducer of MDSCs (Yazawa et al., 2013). The effects of IL-17 may be either direct or indirect. Most cells have IL-17 receptors so MDSCs may be directly impacted. However, IL-17 triggers the production of IL-6 which in turn activates STAT3, so many effects on MDSCs may be directly mediated by IL-6 and indirectly by IL-17 (Chatterjee et al., 2013; Wang et al., 2009).[191]"

Covid-19 raises interleukin 17 levels
Interleukin-17A (IL-17A): A silent amplifier of COVID-19[192]
High Glucose raises interleukin 17 levels
Elevated Interleukin-17 Levels in Patients with Newly Diagnosed Type 2 Diabetes Mellitus[193]
Cannabinoids lower interleukin 17 levels
The Effect of Cannabis on the Clinical and Cytokine Profiles in Patients with Multiple Sclerosis[194]

Curcumin inhibits interleukin 17
Inhibition of interleukin 17 production by curcumin in mice with collagen-induced arthritis[195]

187 Wessam Mustafa, Nadia Elgendy, Samer Salama, Mohamed Jawad, Khaled Eltoukhy, "The Effect of Cannabis on the Clinical and Cytokine Profiles in Patients with Multiple Sclerosis", Multiple Sclerosis International, vol. 2021, Article ID 6611897, 10 pages, 2021. https://doi.org/10.1155/2021/6611897

188 Kang BY, Song YJ, Kim KM, Choe YK, Hwang SY, Kim TS. Curcumin inhibits Th1 cytokine profile in CD4+ T cells by suppressing interleukin-12 production in macrophages. Br J Pharmacol. 1999 Sep;128(2):380-4. doi: 10.1038/sj.bjp.0702803. PMID: 10510448; PMCID: PMC1571646.

189 Ahangar-Parvin, Rayhaneh et al. "The Modulatory Effects of Vitamin D on the Expression of IL-12 and TGF-β in the Spinal Cord and Serum of Mice with Experimental Autoimmune Encephalomyelitis." Iranian journal of pathology vol. 13,1 (2018): 10-22.

190 Reyes-García MG, Hernández-Hernández F, Hernández-Téllez B, García-Tamayo F. GABA (A) receptor subunits RNA expression in mice peritoneal macrophages modulate their IL-6/IL-12 production. J Neuroimmunol. 2007 Aug;188(1-2):64-8. doi: 10.1016/j.jneuroim.2007.05.013. Epub 2007 Jun 27. PMID: 17599468.

191 Katherine H. Parker, ... Suzanne Ostrand-Rosenberg, in Advances in Cancer Research, 2015

192 Francesco Maione, Gian Marco Casillo, Federica Raucci, Cristian Salvatore, Giovanna Ambrosini, Luisa Costa, Raffaele Scarpa, Francesco Caso, Mariarosaria Bucci,Interleukin-17A (IL-17A): A silent amplifier of COVID-19,Biomedicine & Pharmacotherapy,Volume 142,2021,111980,ISSN 0753-3322,https://doi.org/10.1016/j.biopha.2021.111980.

193 Chen C, Shao Y, Wu X, Huang C, Lu W (2016) Elevated Interleukin-17 Levels in Patients with Newly Diagnosed Type 2 Diabetes Mellitus. Biochem Physiol 5:206. doi: 10.4172/2168-9652.1000206

194 Wessam Mustafa, Nadia Elgendy, Samer Salama, Mohamed Jawad, Khaled Eltoukhy, "The Effect of Cannabis on the Clinical and Cytokine Profiles in Patients with Multiple Sclerosis", Multiple Sclerosis International, vol. 2021, Article ID 6611897, 10 pages, 2021. https://doi.org/10.1155/2021/6611897

Vitamin D inhibits interleukin 17
Vitamin D inhibits pro-inflammatory cytokines in the airways of cystic fibrosis patients infected by Pseudomonas aeruginosa- pilot study | Italian Journal of Pediatrics[196]
Gaba: no effect
Inhibitory role for GABA in autoimmune inflammation[197]

30. IL-18 (Interleukin-18)

"IL-18 is a 22-kD proinflammatory cytokine, which increases in the kidney after ischemia-reperfusion injury, glycerol injection, and cisplatin-induced renal injury in a caspase-1–dependent manner.[198]"

Covid-19 raises interleukin-18 levels
Prognostic value of interleukin-18 and its association with other inflammatory markers and disease severity in COVID-19[199]

High Glucose raises interleukin-18 levels
Interleukin-18 serum level is elevated in type 2 diabetes and latent autoimmune diabetes[200]

Cannabinoids lower interleukin-18 levels
Cannabinoids as Key Regulators of Inflammasome Signaling: A Current Perspective[201]

Curcumin lowers production of interleukin 18
Curcumin Suppresses the Production of Pro-inflammatory Cytokine Interleukin-18 in Lipopolysaccharide Stimulated Murine Macrophage-Like Cells[202]

Vitamin D lowers interleukin 18 levels
Relationship between serum 25-hydroxyvitamin D and inflammatory cytokines in paediatric sickle cell disease[203]

Gaba reduces production of interleukin 18
Oral microbe-host interactions: influence of β-glucans on gene expression of inflammatory cytokines and metabolome profile[204]

---

195 Biomedical Research (2011) Volume 22, Issue 3. Inhibition of interleukin 17 production by curcumin in mice with collagen-induced arthritis. Yoshihiro Okamoto*, Mayuri Tanaka, Takashi Fukui, Toshiyuki Masuzawa Laboratory of Immunology and Microbiology, Faculty of Pharmacy, Chiba Institute of Science, 3 Shiomi-cho, Choshi, Chiba 288-0025, Japan

196 Olszowiec-Chlebna, M., Koniarek-Maniecka, A., Brzozowska, A. et al. Vitamin D inhibits pro-inflammatory cytokines in the airways of cystic fibrosis patients infected by Pseudomonas aeruginosa- pilot study. Ital J Pediatr 45, 41 (2019). https://doi.org/10.1186/s13052-019-0634-x

197 Bhat R, Axtell R, Mitra A, Miranda M, Lock C, Tsien RW, Steinman L. Inhibitory role for GABA in autoimmune inflammation. Proc Natl Acad Sci U S A. 2010 Feb 9;107(6):2580-5. doi: 10.1073/pnas.0915139107. Epub 2010 Feb 1. PMID: 20133656; PMCID: PMC2823917.

198 From: Critical Care Nephrology (Third Edition), 2019

199 Hasan SatÄ±ÅŸ, Hasan Selçuk Ã–zger, PÄ±nar Aysert YÄ±ldÄ±z, Kenan HÄ±zel, Ã–zlem Gulbahar, Gonca ErbaÅŸ, GÃ¼lbin Aygencel, Ozlem Guzel Tunccan, Mehmet Akif Ã–ztÃ¼rk, Murat Dizbay, Abdurrahman Tufan, Prognostic value of interleukin-18 and its association with other inflammatory markers and disease severity in COVID-19,Cytokine,Volume 137, 2021,155302,ISSN 1043-4666,https://doi.org/10.1016/j.cyto.2020.155302.

200 Zaharieva, Emanuela et al. "Interleukin-18 serum level is elevated in type 2 diabetes and latent autoimmune diabetes." Endocrine connections vol. 7,1 (2018): 179-185. doi:10.1530/EC-17-0273

201 Suryavanshi Santosh V., Kovalchuk Igor, Kovalchuk Olga. Frontiers in Immunology. Volume 11, 2021

202 Yadav R, Jee B, Awasthi SK. Curcumin Suppresses the Production of Pro-inflammatory Cytokine Interleukin-18 in Lipopolysaccharide Stimulated Murine Macrophage-Like Cells. Indian J Clin Biochem. 2015 Jan;30(1):109-12. doi: 10.1007/s12291-014-0452-2. Epub 2014 Jul 15. PMID: 25646051; PMCID: PMC4310836.

203 Samuel Ademola Adegoke, Olufemi Samuel Smith, Adekunle D. Adekile, Maria Stella Figueiredo, Relationship between serum 25-hydroxyvitamin D and inflammatory cytokines in paediatric sickle cell disease, Cytokine, Volume 96, 2017, Pages 87-93, ISSN 1043-4666, https://doi.org/10.1016/j.cyto.2017.03.010.

31. IL-33 (interleukin-33)

"Interleukin-33 (IL-33) is a tissue-derived nuclear cytokine from the IL-1 family abundantly expressed in endothelial cells, epithelial cells and fibroblast-like cells, both during homeostasis and inflammation. It functions as an alarm signal (alarmin) released upon cell injury or tissue damage to alert immune cells expressing the ST2 receptor (IL-1RL1). The major targets of IL-33 in vivo are tissue-resident immune cells such as mast cells, group 2 innate lymphoid cells (ILC2s) and regulatory T cells (Tregs). Other cellular targets include T helper 2 (Th2) cells, eosinophils, basophils, dendritic cells, Th1 cells, CD8+ T cells, NK cells, iNKT cells, B cells, neutrophils and macrophages. IL-33 is thus emerging as a crucial immune modulator with pleiotropic activities in type-2, type-1 and regulatory immune responses, and important roles in allergic, fibrotic, infectious, and chronic inflammatory diseases."

(*Interleukin-33 (IL-33): A nuclear cytokine from the IL-1 family*[205])

Interleukin 33 levels raised with Covid-19 severity
IL 33 Correlates With COVID-19 Severity, Radiographic and Clinical Finding[206]
High Glucose raises interleukin 33 levels
Circulating levels of IL-33 are elevated by obesity and positively correlated with metabolic disorders in Chinese adults[207]
Cannabinoids normalize levels of interleukin-33
Cannabidiol Ameliorates Cognitive Function via Regulation of IL-33 and TREM2 Upregulation in a Murine Model of Alzheimer's Disease[208]
Curcumin suppresses interleukin-33
The Immunomodulatory and Anti-Inflammatory Effect of Curcumin on Immune Cell Populations, Cytokines, and In Vivo Models of Rheumatoid Arthritis[209]
Vitamin D decreases interleukin-33
Vitamin D Modulates the Expression of IL-27 and IL-33 in the Central Nervous System in Experimental Autoimmune Encephalomyelitis (EAE)[210]
Gaba: no data found

32. IFN-y (interferon gamma/type II interferon)

"IFNγ is a cytokine with important roles in tissue homeostasis, immune and inflammatory responses and tumour immunosurveillance. Signalling by the IFNγ receptor activates the Janus kinase (JAK)-signal transducer and activator of transcription 1 (STAT1) pathway to induce the expression of

204 Silva VO, Pereira LJ, Murata RM. Oral microbe-host interactions: influence of β-glucans on gene expression of inflammatory cytokines and metabolome profile. BMC Microbiol. 2017 Mar 7;17(1):53. doi: 10.1186/s12866-017-0946-1. PMID: 28270109; PMCID: PMC5341410.

205 Cayrol C, Girard JP. Interleukin-33 (IL-33): A nuclear cytokine from the IL-1 family. Immunol Rev. 2018 Jan;281(1):154-168. doi: 10.1111/imr.12619. PMID: 29247993.

206 Markovic Sofija Sekulic, Jovanovic Marina, Gajovic Nevena, Jurisevic Milena, Arsenijevic Nebojsa, Jovanovic Marina, Jovanovic Milan, Mijailovic Zeljko, Lukic Snezana, Zornic Nenad, Vukicevic Vladimir, Stojanovic Jasmina, Maric Veljko, Jocic Miodrag, Jovanovic Ivan. Frontiers in Medicine. Volume 8, 2021. https://www.frontiersin.org/article/10.3389/fmed.2021.749569. DOI=10.3389/fmed.2021.749569. ISSN=2296-858X

207 Tang, Haoneng et al. "Circulating levels of IL-33 are elevated by obesity and positively correlated with metabolic disorders in Chinese adults." Journal of translational medicine vol. 19,1 52. 4 Feb. 2021, doi:10.1186/s12967-021-02711-x

208 Khodadadi H, Salles ÉL, Jarrahi A, Costigliola V, Khan MB, Yu JC, Morgan JC, Hess DC, Vaibhav K, Dhandapani KM, Baban B. Cannabidiol Ameliorates Cognitive Function via Regulation of IL-33 and TREM2 Upregulation in a Murine Model of Alzheimer's Disease. J Alzheimers Dis. 2021;80(3):973-977. doi: 10.3233/JAD-210026. PMID: 33612548.

209 Makuch, Sebastian et al. "The Immunomodulatory and Anti-Inflammatory Effect of Curcumin on Immune Cell Populations, Cytokines, and In Vivo Models of Rheumatoid Arthritis." Pharmaceuticals (Basel, Switzerland) vol. 14,4 309. 1 Apr. 2021, doi:10.3390/ph14040309

210 Mohammadi-Kordkhayli M, Ahangar-Parvin R, Azizi SV, Nemati M, Shamsizadeh A, Khaksari M, Moazzeni SM, Jafarzadeh A. Vitamin D Modulates the Expression of IL-27 and IL-33 in the Central Nervous System in Experimental Autoimmune Encephalomyelitis (EAE). Iran J Immunol. 2015 Mar;12(1):35-49. PMID: 25784096.

classical interferon-stimulated genes that have key immune effector functions. This Review focuses on recent advances in our understanding of the transcriptional, chromatin-based and metabolic mechanisms that underlie IFNγ-mediated polarization of macrophages to an 'M1-like' state, which is characterized by increased pro-inflammatory activity and macrophage resistance to tolerogenic and anti-inflammatory factors. In addition, I describe the newly discovered effects of IFNγ on other leukocytes, vascular cells, adipose tissue cells, neurons and tumour cells that have important implications for autoimmunity, metabolic diseases, atherosclerosis, neurological diseases and immune checkpoint blockade cancer therapy." (*IFNγ: signalling, epigenetics and roles in immunity, metabolism, disease and cancer immunotherapy*[211])

Covid-19 raises IFN-y.
Lower Circulating Interferon-Gamma Is a Risk Factor for Lung Fibrosis in COVID-19 Patients[212]
High Glucose raises IFN-y
High glucose attenuates insulin-induced VEGF expression in bovine retinal microvascular endothelial cells[213]
Cannabinoids lower IFN-y
Combination of Cannabinoids, Δ9- Tetrahydrocannabinol and Cannabidiol, Ameliorates Experimental Multiple Sclerosis by Suppressing Neuroinflammation Through Regulation of miRNA-Mediated Signaling Pathways[214]
Curcumin lowers IFN-y
Curcumin mediates attenuation of pro-inflammatory interferon γ and interleukin 17 cytokine responses in psoriatic disease, strengthening its role as a dietary immunosuppressant[215]
Vitamin D lowers IFN-y
Effect of vitamin D supplementation on cathelicidin, IFN-γ, IL-4 and Th1/Th2 transcription factors in young healthy females[216]
Gaba: no data found

33. TNF/TNF-α (tumor necrosis factor alpha or cachexin, or cachectin)

"Tumour Necrosis Factor alpha (TNF alpha), is an inflammatory cytokine produced by macrophages/monocytes during acute inflammation and is responsible for a diverse range of signalling events within cells, leading to necrosis or apoptosis. The protein is also important for resistance to infection and cancers. TNF alpha exerts many of its effects by binding, as a trimer, to either a 55 kDa cell membrane receptor termed TNFR-1 or a 75 kDa cell membrane receptor termed TNFR-2. Both these receptors belong to the so-called TNF receptor superfamily. The superfamily includes FAS, CD40, CD27, and RANK." (*TNF alpha and the TNF receptor superfamily: structure-function relationship(s). National Library of Medicine, NIH*[217])

211 Ivashkiv LB. IFNγ: signalling, epigenetics and roles in immunity, metabolism, disease and cancer immunotherapy. Nat Rev Immunol. 2018 Sep;18(9):545-558. doi: 10.1038/s41577-018-0029-z. PMID: 29921905; PMCID: PMC6340644.
212 Hu, Zhong-Jie et al. "Lower Circulating Interferon-Gamma Is a Risk Factor for Lung Fibrosis in COVID-19 Patients." Frontiers in immunology vol. 11 585647. 29 Sep. 2020, doi:10.3389/fimmu.2020.585647
213 Wu, H., Xia, X., Jiang, C. et al. High glucose attenuates insulin-induced VEGF expression in bovine retinal microvascular endothelial cells. Eye 24, 145–151 (2010). https://doi.org/10.1038/eye.2009.157
214 Al-Ghezi Zinah Zamil, Miranda Kathryn, Nagarkatti Mitzi, Nagarkatti Prakash S.Combination of Cannabinoids, Î"9-Tetrahydrocannabinol and Cannabidiol, Ameliorates Experimental Multiple Sclerosis by Suppressing Neuroinflammation Through Regulation of miRNA-Mediated Signaling Pathways. Frontiers in Immunology. Volume 10, 2019. https://www.frontiersin.org/article/10.3389/fimmu.2019.01921   DOI=10.3389/fimmu.2019.01921.ISSN=1664-3224
215 Skyvalidas DN, Mavropoulos A, Tsiogkas S, Dardiotis E, Liaskos C, Mamuris Z, Roussaki-Schulze A, Sakkas LI, Zafiriou E, Bogdanos DP. Curcumin mediates attenuation of pro-inflammatory interferon γ and interleukin 17 cytokine responses in psoriatic disease, strengthening its role as a dietary immunosuppressant. Nutr Res. 2020 Mar;75:95-108. doi: 10.1016/j.nutres.2020.01.005. Epub 2020 Feb 27. PMID: 32114280.
216 Das, M., Tomar, N., Sreenivas, V.et al. Effect of vitamin D supplementation on cathelicidin, IFN-γ, IL-4 and Th1/Th2 transcription factors in young healthy females. Eur J Clin Nutr 68, 338–343 (2014). https://doi.org/10.1038/ejcn.2013.268
217 Idriss HT, Naismith JH. TNF alpha and the TNF receptor superfamily: structure-function relationship(s). Microsc Res Tech. 2000 Aug 1;50(3):184-95. doi: 10.1002/1097-0029(20000801)50:3<184::AID-JEMT2>3.0.CO;2-H. PMID: 10891884.

Covid-19 raises TNF-α
Increased Serum Levels of Soluble TNF-α Receptor Is Associated With ICU Mortality in COVID-19 Patients[218]
Dietary Sugars increase TNF-α
Effect of Dietary Sugar Intake on Biomarkers of Subclinical Inflammation: A Systematic Review and Meta-Analysis of Intervention Studies[219]
Cannabinoids reduce TNF-α
The Effects of Cannabinoids on Pro- and Anti-Inflammatory Cytokines: A Systematic Review of In Vivo Studies[220]
Curcumin reduces TNF-α
Curcumin downregulates human tumor necrosis factor-α levels: A systematic review and meta-analysis of randomized controlled trials[221]
Vitamin D reduces TNF-α
Vitamin D and Serum Cytokines in a Randomized Clinical Trial[222]
Gaba enhances TNF-a, but also enhances TNF-b, which counters this effect
Sub-basal increases of GABA enhance the synthesis of TNF-α, TGF-β, and IL-1β in the immune system organs of the Nile tilapia[223]

34. APN/GBP28/apM1 (adiponectin/AdipoQ and Acrp30)

"Adiponectin (APN) is a unique adipokine with multiple salutary effects such as antiapoptotic, anti-inflammatory, and anti-oxidative activities in numerous organs and cells. Chronic obstructive pulmonary disease (COPD), a growing cause of mortality and morbidity worldwide, often results from the smoking habit and is considered a lifestyle-related disease. COPD is frequently complicated with comorbidities, such as cardiovascular disease, diabetes mellitus, and osteoporosis; however, the molecular mechanisms linking COPD and the associated comorbidities are poorly understood. Recent data have revealed a role for APN in the lung; mice lacking APN spontaneously develop a COPD-like phenotype with extrapulmonary effects, including systemic inflammation, body weight loss, and osteoporosis. This finding highlights the key role of APN in lung pathology and the novel cross talk between lung and adipose tissues. [224]."

Covid-19 Lowers Adiponectin

218 Mortaz Esmaeil, Tabarsi Payam, Jamaati Hamidreza, Dalil Roofchayee Neda, Dezfuli Neda K., Hashemian Seyed MohammadReza, Moniri Afshin, Marjani Majid, Malekmohammad Majid, Mansouri Davood, Varahram Mohammad, Folkerts Gert, Adcock Ian M. Increased Serum Levels of Soluble TNF-Î± Receptor Is Associated With ICU Mortality in COVID-19 Patients.Frontiers in Immunology. Volume 12, 2021.
https://www.frontiersin.org/article/10.3389/fimmu.2021.592727 DOI=10.3389/fimmu.2021.592727. ISSN=1664-3224

219 International Journal of Medical Arts. Al-Azhar University (Damietta), Faculty of Medicine. 2636-4174. Taha, Sara I. El Sehsah, Eman M. Fouad, Shaimaa H. Ezzelregal, Hieba G., A Moussa, Aya H. Abdalgeleel, Shaimaa A. Abdelmaksoud, Mariam F. 01/01/2022

220 Henshaw FR, Dewsbury LS, Lim CK, Steiner GZ. The Effects of Cannabinoids on Pro- and Anti-Inflammatory Cytokines: A Systematic Review of In Vivo Studies. Cannabis Cannabinoid Res. 2021 Jun;6(3):177-195. doi: 10.1089/can.2020.0105. Epub 2021 Apr 28. PMID: 33998900; PMCID: PMC8266561.

221 Sahebkar A, Cicero AFG, Simental-Mendía LE, Aggarwal BB, Gupta SC. Curcumin downregulates human tumor necrosis factor-α levels: A systematic review and meta-analysis of randomized controlled trials. Pharmacol Res. 2016 May;107:234-242. doi: 10.1016/j.phrs.2016.03.026. Epub 2016 Mar 26. PMID: 27025786.

222 Eleanor Yusupov, Melissa Li-Ng, Simcha Pollack, James K. Yeh, Mageda Mikhail, John F. Aloia, "Vitamin D and Serum Cytokines in a Randomized Clinical Trial", International Journal of Endocrinology, vol. 2010, Article ID 305054, 7 pages, 2010. https://doi.org/10.1155/2010/305054

223 Nájera-Martínez M, López-Tapia BP, Aguilera-Alvarado GP, Madera-Sandoval RL, Sánchez-Nieto S, Giron-Pérez MI, Vega-López A. Sub-basal increases of GABA enhance the synthesis of TNF-α, TGF-β, and IL-1β in the immune system organs of the Nile tilapia. J Neuroimmunol. 2020 Nov 15;348:577382. doi: 10.1016/j.jneuroim.2020.577382. Epub 2020 Sep 4. PMID: 32919148.

224 Takeda Y, Nakanishi K, Tachibana I, Kumanogoh A. Adiponectin: a novel link between adipocytes and COPD. Vitam Horm. 2012;90:419-35. doi: 10.1016/B978-0-12-398313-8.00016-6. PMID: 23017725.

Hyperglycemia in acute COVID-19 is characterized by insulin resistance and adipose tissue infectivity by SARS-CoV-2[225]

High Adiponectin Lowers Blood Sugar

Adiponectin, a Therapeutic Target for Obesity, Diabetes, and Endothelial Dysfunction[226]

Cannabinoids Increase Adiponectin Levels

Efficacy and Safety of Cannabidioland Tetrahydrocannabivarin on Glycemic and Lipid Parameters inPatients With Type 2 Diabetes: ARandomized, Double-Blind,Placebo-Controlled, Parallel GroupPilot Study[227]

Curcumin Increases Adiponectin Levels

The effect of curcumin supplementation on circulating adiponectin: A systematic review and meta-analysis of randomized controlled trials[228]

Vitamin D Increases Adiponectin Levels

The effect of vitamin D supplementation on insulin resistance, visceral fat and adiponectin in vitamin D deficient women with polycystic ovary syndrome: a randomized placebo-controlled trial[229]

Gaba Increases Adiponectin Levels

Oral administration of γ-aminobutyric acid and γ-oryzanol prevents stress-induced hypoadiponectinemia[230]

Regulates gene expression

35. AHR (aryl hydrocarbon receptor)

"The aryl hydrocarbon receptor (AhR) is a cytoplasmic receptor and transcription factor activated through cognate ligand binding. It is an important factor in immunity and tissue homeostasis, and structurally diverse compounds from the environment, diet, microbiome, and host metabolism can induce AhR activity. Emerging evidence suggests that AhR is a key sensor allowing immune cells to adapt to environmental conditions and changes in AhR activity have been associated with autoimmune disorders and cancer. Furthermore, AhR

225 Reiterer M, Rajan M, Gómez-Banoy N, Lau JD, Gomez-Escobar LG, Ma L, Gilani A, Alvarez-Mulett S, Sholle ET, Chandar V, Bram Y, Hoffman K, Bhardwaj P, Piloco P, Rubio-Navarro A, Uhl S, Carrau L, Houhgton S, Redmond D, Shukla AP, Goyal P, Brown KA, tenOever BR, Alonso LC, Schwartz RE, Schenck EJ, Safford MM, Lo JC. Hyperglycemia in acute COVID-19 is characterized by insulin resistance and adipose tissue infectivity by SARS-CoV-2. Cell Metab. 2021 Nov 2;33(11):2174-2188.e5. doi: 10.1016/j.cmet.2021.09.009. Epub 2021 Sep 16. Erratum in: Cell Metab. 2021 Dec 7;33(12):2484. PMID: 34599884; PMCID: PMC8443335.

226 Achari AE, Jain SK. Adiponectin, a Therapeutic Target for Obesity, Diabetes, and Endothelial Dysfunction. Int J Mol Sci. 2017 Jun 21;18(6):1321. doi: 10.3390/ijms18061321. PMID: 28635626; PMCID: PMC5486142.

227 Jadoon KA, Ratcliffe SH, Barrett DA, Thomas EL, Stott C, Bell JD, O'Sullivan SE, Tan GD. Efficacy and Safety of Cannabidiol and Tetrahydrocannabivarin on Glycemic and Lipid Parameters in Patients With Type 2 Diabetes: A Randomized, Double-Blind, Placebo-Controlled, Parallel Group Pilot Study. Diabetes Care. 2016 Oct;39(10):1777-86. doi: 10.2337/dc16-0650. Epub 2016 Aug 29. PMID: 27573936.

228 Clark CCT, Ghaedi E, Arab A, Pourmasoumi M, Hadi A. The effect of curcumin supplementation on circulating adiponectin: A systematic review and meta-analysis of randomized controlled trials. Diabetes Metab Syndr. 2019 Sep-Oct;13(5):2819-2825. doi: 10.1016/j.dsx.2019.07.045. Epub 2019 Jul 30. PMID: 31425942.

229 Seyyed Abootorabi M, Ayremlou P, Behroozi-Lak T, Nourisaeidlou S. The effect of vitamin D supplementation on insulin resistance, visceral fat and adiponectin in vitamin D deficient women with polycystic ovary syndrome: a randomized placebo-controlled trial. Gynecol Endocrinol. 2018 Jun;34(6):489-494. doi: 10.1080/09513590.2017.1418311. Epub 2017 Dec 22. Erratum in: Gynecol Endocrinol. 2018 Sep;34(9):740. PMID: 29271278.

230 Ohara K, Kiyotani Y, Uchida A, Nagasaka R, Maehara H, Kanemoto S, Hori M, Ushio H. Oral administration of γ-aminobutyric acid and γ-oryzanol prevents stress-induced hypoadiponectinemia. Phytomedicine. 2011 Jun 15;18(8-9):655-60. doi: 10.1016/j.phymed.2011.01.003. Epub 2011 Feb 11. PMID: 21316207.

agonists or antagonists can impact immune disease outcomes identifying AhR as a potentially actionable target for immunotherapy.[231]"

Covid-19 induces AHR signaling
AHR signaling is induced by infection with coronaviruses[232]

Glucose activates AHR
Aryl Hydrocarbon Receptor (AhR) is Activated by Glucose and Regulates the Thrombospondin-1 Gene Promoter in Endothelial Cells[233]

Cannabinoids reduce AHR activation
Role of Epigenome and Microbiome in Cannabinoid and Aryl Hydrocarbon Receptor-Mediated Regulation of Inflammatory and Autoimmune Diseases[234]

Curcumin suppresses AHR activation
Effect of Curcumin on the Aryl Hydrocarbon Receptor and Cytochrome P450 1A1 in MCF-7 Human Breast Carcinoma Cells[235]

Vitamin D suppresses AHR activation
AhR is a molecular target of Calcitriol in human T cells[236]
Gaba: *No data found*

Cytokine activation

36. CASP1/ICE (Caspase-1/Interleukin-1 converting enzyme)
"This gene encodes a protein which is a member of the cysteine-aspartic acid protease (caspase) family. Sequential activation of caspases plays a central role in the execution-phase of cell apoptosis. Caspases exist as inactive proenzymes which undergo proteolytic processing at conserved aspartic residues to produce 2 subunits, large and small, that dimerize to form the active enzyme. This gene was identified by its ability to proteolytically cleave and activate the inactive precursor of interleukin-1, a cytokine involved in the processes such as inflammation, septic shock, and wound healing."
(*CASP1. National Library of Medicine, NIH*)

Covid-19 activates CASP1
SARS-CoV-2 engages inflammasome and pyroptosis in human primary monocytes[237]

Glucose stimulates CASP1
Purinergic regulation of high-glucose-induced caspase-1 activation in the rat retinal Müller cell line rMC-1[238]

231 Shinde R, McGaha TL. The Aryl Hydrocarbon Receptor: Connecting Immunity to the Microenvironment. Trends Immunol. 2018 Dec;39(12):1005-1020. doi: 10.1016/j.it.2018.10.010. Epub 2018 Nov 5. PMID: 30409559; PMCID: PMC7182078.

232 Giovannoni, F., Li, Z., Remes-Lenicov, F. et al. AHR signaling is induced by infection with coronaviruses. Nat Commun 12, 5148 (2021). https://doi.org/10.1038/s41467-021-25412-x

233 Dabir, Pankaj et al. "Aryl hydrocarbon receptor is activated by glucose and regulates the thrombospondin-1 gene promoter in endothelial cells." Circulation research vol. 102,12 (2008): 1558-65. doi:10.1161/CIRCRESAHA.108.176990

234 Al-Ghezi, Z. Z.(2019). Role of Epigenome and Microbiome in Cannabinoid and Aryl Hydrocarbon Receptor-Mediated Regulation of Inflammatory and Autoimmune Diseases. (Doctoral dissertation). Retrieved from https://scholarcommons.sc.edu/etd/5342

235 Ciolino HP, Daschner PJ, Wang TT, Yeh GC. Effect of curcumin on the aryl hydrocarbon receptor and cytochrome P450 1A1 in MCF-7 human breast carcinoma cells. Biochem Pharmacol. 1998 Jul 15;56(2):197-206. doi: 10.1016/s0006-2952(98)00143-9. PMID: 9698073.

236 Takami, Mariko et al. "Cutting Edge: AhR Is a Molecular Target of Calcitriol in Human T Cells." Journal of immunology (Baltimore, Md. : 1950) vol. 195,6 (2015): 2520-3. doi:10.4049/jimmunol.1500344

237 Ferreira, A.C., Soares, V.C., de Azevedo-Quintanilha, I.G. et al. SARS-CoV-2 engages inflammasome and pyroptosis in human primary monocytes. Cell Death Discov. 7, 43 (2021). https://doi.org/10.1038/s41420-021-00428-w

238 Trueblood KE, Mohr S, Dubyak GR. Purinergic regulation of high-glucose-induced caspase-1 activation in the rat retinal Müller cell line rMC-1. Am J Physiol Cell Physiol. 2011 Nov;301(5):C1213-23. doi: 10.1152/ajpcell.00265.2011. Epub 2011 Aug 10. PMID: 21832250; PMCID: PMC3213916.

Cannabinoids decrease CASP1
Cannabinoids as Key Regulators of Inflammasome Signaling: A Current Perspective[239]
Curcumin inhibits CASP1
Curcumin Suppresses IL-1β Secretion and Prevents Inflammation through Inhibition of the NLRP3 Inflammasome[240]
Vitamin D deficiency activates CASP1
Vitamin D Receptor Inhibits NLRP3 Activation by Impeding Its BRCC3-Mediated Deubiquitination[241]
Gaba: no data found

37. MyD88

"MYD88 is an adaptor protein that interacts with IRAK4 and IRAK1 to activate both the NFκB and interferon pathways through TRAF6."[242]
COVID-19 raises MyD88, but it lowers close to septic shock
Myeloid phenotypes in severe COVID-19 predict secondary infection and mortality: a pilot study
MyD88 deficiency worsens Covid-19
Varying Illness Severity in Patients with MyD88 Deficiency Infected with Coronavirus SARS-CoV-2[243]
Fructose raises MyD88
Toll-like receptors 1–9 are elevated in livers with fructose-induced hepatic steatosis[244]
MyD88 signaling is increased in obesity
Increased TLR/MyD88 signaling in patients with obesity: is there a link to COVID-19 disease severity?[245]
Cannabinoids reduce MyD88 release by inhibiting TLR3 and TLR4
MyD88-dependent and -independent signalling via TLR3 and TLR4 are differentially modulated by Δ9-tetrahydrocannabinol and cannabidiol in human macrophages[246]
Curcumin inhibits MyD88 via TLR4
Curcumin attenuates acute inflammatory injury by inhibiting the TLR4/MyD88/NF-κB signaling pathway in experimental traumatic brain injury

239 Suryavanshi, Santosh V et al. "Cannabinoids as Key Regulators of Inflammasome Signaling: A Current Perspective." Frontiers in immunology vol. 11 613613. 28 Jan. 2021, doi:10.3389/fimmu.2020.613613

240 Yin H, Guo Q, Li X, Tang T, Li C, Wang H, Sun Y, Feng Q, Ma C, Gao C, Yi F, Peng J. Curcumin Suppresses IL-1β Secretion and Prevents Inflammation through Inhibition of the NLRP3 Inflammasome. J Immunol. 2018 Apr 15;200(8):2835-2846. doi: 10.4049/jimmunol.1701495. Epub 2018 Mar 16. PMID: 29549176.

241 Rao, Zebing et al. "Vitamin D Receptor Inhibits NLRP3 Activation by Impeding Its BRCC3-Mediated Deubiquitination." Frontiers in immunology vol. 10 2783. 4 Dec. 2019, doi:10.3389/fimmu.2019.02783

242 From: The Molecular Basis of Cancer (Fourth Edition), 2015

243 Mahmood, Hera Z. et al. "Varying Illness Severity in Patients with MyD88 Deficiency Infected with Coronavirus SARS-CoV-2." (2021).

244 Wagnerberger, S., Spruss, A., Kanuri, G., Volynets, V., Stahl, C., Bischoff, S., & Bergheim, I. (2012). Toll-like receptors 1–9 are elevated in livers with fructose-induced hepatic steatosis. British Journal of Nutrition, 107(12), 1727-1738. doi:10.1017/S0007114511004983

245 Cuevas AM, Clark JM, Potter JJ. Increased TLR/MyD88 signaling in patients with obesity: is there a link to COVID-19 disease severity? Int J Obes (Lond). 2021 May;45(5):1152-1154. doi: 10.1038/s41366-021-00768-8. Epub 2021 Feb 26. PMID: 33637950; PMCID: PMC7909368.

246 John-Mark Fitzpatrick, Eleanor Minogue, Lucy Curham, Harry Tyrrell, Philip Gavigan, William Hind, Eric J. Downer, MyD88-dependent and -independent signalling via TLR3 and TLR4 are differentially modulated by Δ9 tetrahydrocannabinol and cannabidiol in human macrophages, Journal of Neuroimmunology, Volume 343,2020,577217,ISSN 0165-5728, https://doi.org/10.1016/j.jneuroim.2020.577217. (https://www.sciencedirect.com/science/article/pii/S0165572820300576)

Vitamin D down-regulates genes related to MyD88
Gene expression analysis reveals vitamin D regulates genes critical to oncogenesis in MYD88 mutated B cell lymphomas.[247]
Gaba inhibits MyD88
<u>**Effects of dietary gamma-aminobutyric acid supplementation on the intestinal functions in weaning piglets**</u>[248]

Blood Coagulation and Angiogenesis

38. ANGIOGENESIS (NEW BLOOD VESSLE GROWTH)
Angiogenesis is raised by Covid-19
Pulmonary Vascular Endothelialitis, Thrombosis, and Angiogenesis in Covid-19[249]
High Glucose causes aberrant angiogenesis
Novel Tissue-Specific Mechanism of Regulation of Angiogenesis and Cancer Growth in Response to Hyperglycemia[250]
Cannabinoids suppress angiogenesis
Endocannabinoids as emerging suppressors of angiogenesis and tumor invasion (Review)[251]
Cannabidiol inhibits angiogenesis by multiple mechanisms[252]
Curcumin inhibits angiogenesis
Curcumin as an inhibitor of angiogenesis[253]
Vitamin D inhibits angiogenesis
A systematic review on vitamin d and angiogenesis[254]
Inducing angiogenesis reduces Gaba in mouse brain
<u>*Carnosine and L-arginine attenuate the downregulation of brain monoamines and gamma aminobutyric acid; reverse apoptosis and upregulate the expression of angiogenic factors in a model of hemic hypoxia in rats*</u>[255]

---

247 Tyler Kalajian, Arash Hossein-Nezhad, Michael Holick, Gene expression analysis reveals vitamin D regulates genes critical to oncogenesis in MYD88 mutated B cell lymphomas., Clinical Lymphoma Myeloma and Leukemia, Volume 19, Issue 10, Supplement, 2019, Pages e319-e320, ISSN 2152-2650, https://doi.org/10.1016/j.clml.2019.09.525.

248 Chen S , Tan B , Xia Y , Liao S , Wang M , Yin J , Wang J , Xiao H , Qi M , Bin P , Liu G , Ren W , Yin Y . Effects of dietary gamma-aminobutyric acid supplementation on the intestinal functions in weaning piglets. Food Funct. 2019 Jan 22;10(1):366-378. doi: 10.1039/c8fo02161a. PMID: 30601517.

249 Ackermann M, Verleden SE, Kuehnel M, Haverich A, Welte T, Laenger F, Vanstapel A, Werlein C, Stark H, Tzankov A, Li WW, Li VW, Mentzer SJ, Jonigk D. Pulmonary Vascular Endothelialitis, Thrombosis, and Angiogenesis in Covid-19. N Engl J Med. 2020 Jul 9;383(2):120-128. doi: 10.1056/NEJMoa2015432. Epub 2020 May 21. PMID: 32437596; PMCID: PMC7412750.

250 Bhattacharyya S, Sul K, Krukovets I, Nestor C, Li J, Adognravi OS. Novel tissue-specific mechanism of regulation of angiogenesis and cancer growth in response to hyperglycemia. J Am Heart Assoc. 2012 Dec;1(6):e005967. doi: 10.1161/JAHA.112.005967. Epub 2012 Dec 19. PMID: 23316333; PMCID: PMC3540668.

251 Bifulco M, Laezza C, Gazzerro P, Pentimalli F. Endocannabinoids as emerging suppressors of angiogenesis and tumor invasion (review). Oncol Rep. 2007 Apr;17(4):813-6. PMID: 17342320.

252 Solinas, M et al. "Cannabidiol inhibits angiogenesis by multiple mechanisms." British journal of pharmacology vol. 167,6 (2012): 1218-31. doi:10.1111/j.1476-5381.2012.02050.x

253 Bhandarkar SS, Arbiser JL. Curcumin as an inhibitor of angiogenesis. Adv Exp Med Biol. 2007;595:185-95. doi: 10.1007/978-0-387-46401-5_7. PMID: 17569211.

254 Aliashrafi S, Ebrahimi-Mameghani M7: A SYSTEMATIC REVIEW ON VITAMIN D AND ANGIOGENESISBMJ Open 2017;7:bmjopen-2016-015415.7. doi: 10.1136/bmjopen-2016-015415.7

255 Attia H, Fadda L, Al-Rasheed N, Al-Rasheed N, Maysarah N. Carnosine and L-arginine attenuate the downregulation of brain monoamines and gamma aminobutyric acid; reverse apoptosis and upregulate the expression of angiogenic factors in a model of hemic hypoxia in rats. Naunyn Schmiedebergs Arch Pharmacol. 2020 Mar;393(3):381-394. doi: 10.1007/s00210-019-01738-8. Epub 2019 Oct 22. PMID: 31641819.

39. SEPSIS (BLOOD INFECTION)

"Sepsis is a clinical syndrome defined by a systemic response to infection. With progression to sepsis-associated organ failure (ie, severe sepsis) or hypotension (ie, septic shock) mortality increases. Sepsis is a cause of considerable mortality, morbidity, cost, and health care utilization. Abnormalities in the inflammation, immune, coagulation, oxygen delivery, and utilization pathways play a role in organ dysfunction and death.[256]"

Covid-19 can cause sepsis
COVID-19 and Sepsis[257]
Hyperglycemia increases risk of sepsis
Hyperglycemia in sepsis is a risk factor for development of type II diabetes[258]

Cannabinoids potentially treat sepsis
Cannabis Sativa Revisited—Crosstalk between microRNA Expression, Inflammation, Oxidative Stress, and Endocannabinoid Response System in Critically Ill Patients with Sepsis[259](Preprint)
Cannabidiol Inhibits the Pore-Forming Activity of Gasdermin D in Sepsis [260](preprint)
Curcumin can potentially treat sepsis
Therapeutic effects of curcumin on sepsis and mechanisms of action: A systematic review of preclinical studies[261]
Vitamin D can improve sepsis outcomes
The Correlation between Serum Level of Vitamin D and Outcome of Sepsis Patients; a Cross-Sectional Study[262]
Gaba levels are slightly elevated in Sepsis, but it is unlikely to play a role
Gamma-Aminobutyric Acid (GABA) and Sepsis-Related Encephalopathy[263]

40. VEGF-A,B,C,D/VFP (Vascular endothelial growth factor-a/ vascular permeability factor)

"Vascular endothelial growth factor (VEGF) represents a growth factor with important pro-angiogenic activity, having a mitogenic and an anti-apoptotic effect on endothelial cells, increasing the vascular

256 O'Brien JM Jr, Ali NA, Aberegg SK, Abraham E. Sepsis. Am J Med. 2007 Dec;120(12):1012-22. doi: 10.1016/j.amjmed.2007.01.035. PMID: 18060918.

257 Koçak Tufan Z, Kayaaslan B, Mer M. COVID-19 and Sepsis. Turk J Med Sci. 2021 Dec 17;51(SI-1):3301-3311. doi: 10.3906/sag-2108-239. PMID: 34590796; PMCID: PMC8771020.

258 Gornik, Ivan & Vujaklija Brajković, Ana & Lukić, Edita & Madžarac, Goran & Gasparović, Vladimir. (2009). Hyperglycemia in sepsis is a risk factor for development of type II diabetes. Journal of critical care. 25. 263-9. 10.1016/j.jcrc.2009.10.002.

259 Dinu AR, Rogobete AF, Bratu T, Popovici SE, Bedreag OH, Papurica M, Bratu LM, Sandesc D. Cannabis Sativa Revisited—Crosstalk between microRNA Expression, Inflammation, Oxidative Stress, and Endocannabinoid Response System in Critically Ill Patients with Sepsis. Cells. 2020; 9(2):307. https://doi.org/10.3390/cells9020307

260 Cannabidiol Inhibits the Pore-Forming Activity of Gasdermin D in Sepsis. Posted: 8 Nov 2021. Zhaozheng Li, Central South University - Department of Hematology and Critical Care Medicine, Xiangyu Wang, Central South University - Department of Hematology and Critical Care Medicine, Yang Bai, Central South University - Department of Hematology and Critical Care Medicine, Ling Li, Central South University - Department of Hematology and Critical Care Medicine, Junmei Li, Central South University - Department of Hematology and Critical Care Medicine, Rui Zhang, Central South University - Department of Hematology and Critical Care Medicine, Yiting Tang Central South University, School of Basic Medical Science, Department of Physiology

261 Karimi A, Ghodsi R, Kooshki F, Karimi M, Asghariazar V, Tarighat-Esfanjani A. Therapeutic effects of curcumin on sepsis and mechanisms of action: A systematic review of preclinical studies. Phytother Res. 2019 Nov;33(11):2798-2820. doi: 10.1002/ptr.6467. Epub 2019 Aug 19. PMID: 31429161.

262 Shojaei, Majid et al. "The Correlation between Serum Level of Vitamin D and Outcome of Sepsis Patients; a Cross-Sectional Study." Archives of academic emergency medicine vol. 7,1 e1. 10 Jan. 2019

263 Winder, T., Minuk, G., Sargeant, E., & Seland, T. (1988). Gamma-Aminobutyric Acid (GABA) and Sepsis-Related Encephalopathy. Canadian Journal of Neurological Sciences / Journal Canadien Des Sciences Neurologiques, 15(1), 23-25. doi:10.1017/S0317167100027128

permeability, promoting cell migration, etc. Due to these effects, it actively contributes in regulating the normal and pathological angiogenic processes. In humans, the VEGF family is composed of several members: VEGF-A (which has different isoforms), VEGF-B, VEGF-C, VEGF-D, VEGF-E (viral VEGF), VEGF-F (snake venom VEGF), placenta growth factor (PlGF), and, recently, to this family has been added endocrine gland-derived vascular endothelial growth factor (EG-VEGF)."(**Role of vascular endothelial growth factor in the regulation of angiogenesis**[264]

COVID-19 VEGF changes contribute to illness
The impact of the hypoxia-VEGF-vascular permeability on COVID-19-infected patients[265]
SARS-Covid-19-2 spike protein uses VEGF-A receptor
SARS-CoV-2 Spike protein co-opts VEGF-A/Neuropilin-1 receptor signaling to induce analgesia [266](Preprint)
VEGF-B levels unchanged in COVID-19
COVID-19 is a systemic vascular hemopathy: insight for mechanistic and clinical aspects
VEGF-C levels unchanged in COVID-19
SARS-CoV-2 spike spurs intestinal inflammation via VEGF production in enterocytes
COVID-19 raises VEGF-D levels
VEGF-D: a novel biomarker for detection of COVID-19 progression[267]
High Glucose raises VEGF-A, B
Glucose, VEGF-A, and diabetic complications[268]
Cannabinoids inhibit the VEGF pathway; VEGF-A, B
Cannabinoids Inhibit the Vascular Endothelial Growth Factor Pathway in Gliomas[269]
Cannabinoids and VEGF-D: no data found
Curcumin inhibits VEGF, VEGF-A
Curcumin inhibits VEGF-mediated angiogenesis in human intestinal microvascular endothelial cells through COX-2 and MAPK inhibition[270]
Vitamin D decreases VEGF A, B, C, D
Vitamin D Decreases Serum VEGF Correlating with Clinical Improvement in Vitamin D-Deficient Women with PCOS: A Randomized Placebo-Controlled Trial[271]
VEGF enhances Gaba
VEGF modulates synaptic activity in the developing spinal cord[272]

---

264 Melincovici CS, Boşca AB, Şuşman S, Mărginean M, Mihu C, Istrate M, Moldovan IM, Roman AL, Mihu CM. Vascular endothelial growth factor (VEGF) - key factor in normal and pathological angiogenesis. Rom J Morphol Embryol. 2018;59(2):455-467. PMID: 30173249.

265 Cao Y. The impact of the hypoxia-VEGF-vascular permeability on COVID-19-infected patients. Exploration (Beijing). 2021 Oct;1(2):20210051. doi: 10.1002/EXP.20210051. Epub 2021 Oct 30. PMID: 35434726; PMCID: PMC8653011.

266 Moutal A, Martin LF, Boinon L, Gomez K, Ran D, Zhou Y, Stratton HJ, Cai S, Luo S, Gonzalez KB, Perez-Miller S, Patwardhan A, Ibrahim MM, Khanna R. SARS-CoV-2 Spike protein co-opts VEGF-A/Neuropilin-1 receptor signaling to induce analgesia. bioRxiv [Preprint]. 2020 Sep 14:2020.07.17.209288. doi: 10.1101/2020.07.17.209288. Update in: Pain. 2021 Jan;162(1):243-252. PMID: 32869019; PMCID: PMC7457601.

267 Kong, Y., Han, J., Wu, X. et al. VEGF-D: a novel biomarker for detection of COVID-19 progression. Crit Care 24, 373 (2020). https://doi.org/10.1186/s13054-020-03079-y

268 Benjamin LE. Glucose, VEGF-A, and diabetic complications. Am J Pathol. 2001 Apr;158(4):1181-4. doi: 10.1016/S0002-9440(10)64066-7. PMID: 11290533; PMCID: PMC1891912.

269 Cristina Blázquez, Luis González-Feria, Luis Álvarez, Amador Haro, M. Llanos Casanova, Manuel Guzmán; Cannabinoids Inhibit the Vascular Endothelial Growth Factor Pathway in Gliomas. Cancer Res 15 August 2004; 64 (16): 5617–5623. https://doi.org/10.1158/0008-5472.CAN-03-3927

270 Binion DG, Otterson MF, Rafiee P. Curcumin inhibits VEGF-mediated angiogenesis in human intestinal microvascular endothelial cells through COX-2 and MAPK inhibition. Gut. 2008 Nov;57(11):1509-17. doi: 10.1136/gut.2008.152496. Epub 2008 Jul 2. PMID: 18596194; PMCID: PMC2582343.

271 Irani M, Seifer DB, Grazi RV, Irani S, Rosenwaks Z, Tal R. Vitamin D Decreases Serum VEGF Correlating with Clinical Improvement in Vitamin D-Deficient Women with PCOS: A Randomized Placebo-Controlled Trial. Nutrients. 2017 Mar 28;9(4):334. doi: 10.3390/nu9040334. PMID: 28350328; PMCID: PMC5409673.

272 Guérit S, Allain AE, Léon C, Cazenave W, Ferrara N, Branchereau P, Bikfalvi A. VEGF modulates synaptic activity in the developing spinal cord. Dev Neurobiol. 2014 Nov;74(11):1110-22. doi: 10.1002/dneu.22187. Epub 2014 May 24. PMID: 24782305.

41. PAI-1/serpin E1 (Plasminogen activator inhibitor-1/endothelial plasminogen activator inhibitor)

"Plasminogen activator inhibitor-1 (PAI-1) is a member of the superfamily of serine-protease inhibitors (or serpins), and the principal inhibitor of both the tissue-type and the urokinase-type plasminogen activator, the two plasminogen activators able to activate plasminogen. Current evidence describing the central role played by PAI-1 in a number of age-related subclinical (i.e., inflammation, atherosclerosis, insulin resistance) and clinical (i.e., obesity, comorbidities, Werner syndrome) conditions is presented." (*Plasminogen activator inhibitor-1 (PAI-1): a key factor linking fibrinolysis and age-related subclinical and clinical conditions[273]*)

Covid-19 raises PAI-1
Trapped Inflammatory Molecules Contribute to Long COVID[274]
PAI-1 is elevated in the treatment of diabetes
Effect of plasminogen activator inhibitor-1 in diabetes mellitus and cardiovascular disease[275]
Cannabinoids decrease PAI-1 secretion
Cannabinoids Inhibit the Vascular Endothelial Growth Factor Pathway in Gliomas[276]
Curcumin down-regulates PAI-1
Curcumin Down-Regulates Cytokine-Mediated Tissue Factor and Plasminogen Activator Type 1 Expression In Human Endothelial Cells[277]
Vitamin D down-regulates PAI-1
Vitamin D analogs down-regulate plasminogen activator inhibitor-1 in human coronary artery smooth muscle cell[278]
Gaba: no data found

42. CD4/CD8 (cluster of differentiation 4,8/ cluster of cluster of designation 4,8)

"CD4 is a membrane glycoprotein and a member of the immunoglobulin supergene family and a co-receptor in MHC class II-restricted T-cell activation [5, 48]. It also plays a role in the differentiation of thymocytes and the regulation of T-lymphocyte/B-lymphocyte adhesion [[279]]"

Covid-19 increases CD4 and CD8
Severe COVID-19 is associated with deep and sustained multifaceted cellular immunosuppression[280]
Glucose raises CD4, lowers CD8
Impact of Glucose Loading on Variations in CD4+ and CD8+ T Cells in Japanese Participants with or without Type 2 Diabetes[281]

273 Cesari M, Pahor M, Incalzi RA. Plasminogen activator inhibitor-1 (PAI-1): a key factor linking fibrinolysis and age-related subclinical and clinical conditions. Cardiovasc Ther. 2010 Oct;28(5):e72-91. doi: 10.1111/j.1755-5922.2010.00171.x. Epub 2010 Jul 7. PMID: 20626406; PMCID: PMC2958211.

274 Roni Dengler, PhD. The Scientist. Nov 9, 2021

275 Lyon CJ, Hsueh WA. Effect of plasminogen activator inhibitor-1 in diabetes mellitus and cardiovascular disease. Am J Med. 2003 Dec 8;115 Suppl 8A:62S-68S. doi: 10.1016/j.amjmed.2003.08.014. PMID: 14678868.

276 Cristina Blázquez, Luis González-Feria, Luis Álvarez, Amador Haro, M. Llanos Casanova, Manuel Guzmán; Cannabinoids Inhibit the Vascular Endothelial Growth Factor Pathway in Gliomas. Cancer Res 15 August 2004; 64 (16): 5617–5623. https://doi.org/10.1158/0008-5472.CAN-03-3927

277 Eriko Morishita, Keiko Maruyama, Hidesaku Asakura, Shigeki Ohtake, Akihiro Yachie, Shinji Nakao; Curcumin Down-Regulates Cytokine-Mediated Tissue Factor and Plasminogen Activator Type 1 Expression In Human Endothelial Cells. Blood 2010; 116 (21): 3333. doi: https://doi.org/10.1182/blood.V116.21.3333.3333

278 RUTH WU-WONG, J., NAKANE, M., MA, J. and COOK, A.L. (2005), Vitamin D analogs down-regulate plasminogen activator inhibitor-1 in human coronary artery smooth muscle cells. Journal of Thrombosis and Haemostasis, 3: 1545-1546. https://doi.org/10.1111/j.1538-7836.2005.01459.x

279 Faramarz Naeim, in Hematopathology, 2008

280 Jeannet, R., Daix, T., Formento, R. et al. Severe COVID-19 is associated with deep and sustained multifaceted cellular immunosuppression. Intensive Care Med 46, 1769–1771 (2020). https://doi.org/10.1007/s00134-020-06127-x

281 Miya A, Nakamura A, Miyoshi H, Takano Y, Sunagoya K, Hayasaka K, Shimizu C, Terauchi Y, Atsumi T. Impact of Glucose Loading on Variations in CD4+ and CD8+ T Cells in Japanese Participants with or without Type 2 Diabetes. Front Endocrinol (Lausanne). 2018 Mar 20;9:81. doi: 10.3389/fendo.2018.00081. PMID: 29615971; PMCID: PMC5870166.

Cannabinoids reduce CD4
Effects of Cannabinoids on T-cell Function and Resistance to Infection[282]
Cannabinoids reduce CD8
Heavy Cannabis Use Associated With Reduction in Activated and Inflammatory Immune Cell Frequencies in Antiretroviral Therapy–Treated Human Immunodeficiency Virus–Infected Individuals[283]
Curcumin inhibits CD4 activation
Curcumin Inhibits CD4+ T Cell Activation, but Augments CD69 Expression and TGF-β1-Mediated Generation of Regulatory T Cells at Late Phase[284]
Vitamin D suppresses CD4 and CD8
Vitamin D receptor expression controls proliferation of naïve CD8+ T cells and development of CD8 mediated gastrointestinal inflammation[285]
Gaba inhibits CD4, modulates CD8
γ-Aminobutyric Acid Inhibits T Cell Autoimmunity and the Development of Inflammatory Responses in a Mouse Type 1 Diabetes Model[286]

43. CD142/TF (tissue factor/platelet tissue factor/factor III)

"Under pathological conditions, TF can trigger both arterial and venous thrombosis. For instance, atherosclerotic plaques contain high levels of TF on macrophage foam cells and microvesicles that drives thrombus formation after plaque rupture. In sepsis, inducible TF expression on monocytes leads to disseminated intravascular coagulation." *(American Heart Association Journal)*

Covid-19 elevates TF activity
Patients With COVID-19 Have Elevated Levels of Circulating Extracellular Vesicle Tissue Factor Activity That Is Associated With Severity and Mortality—Brief Report[287]
TF expression raised with High Glucose
Tissue factor expression in obese type 2 diabetic subjects and its regulation by antidiabetic agents[288]

---

282 Eisenstein, Toby K, and Joseph J Meissler. "Effects of Cannabinoids on T-cell Function and Resistance to Infection." Journal of neuroimmune pharmacology : the official journal of the Society on NeuroImmune Pharmacology vol. 10,2 (2015): 204-16. doi:10.1007/s11481-015-9603-3

283 Jennifer A Manuzak, Toni M Gott, Jay S Kirkwood, Ernesto Coronado, Tiffany Hensley-McBain, Charlene Miller, Ryan K Cheu, Ann C Collier, Nicholas T Funderburg, Jeffery N Martin, Michael C Wu, Nina Isoherranen, Peter W Hunt, Nichole R Klatt, Heavy Cannabis Use Associated With Reduction in Activated and Inflammatory Immune Cell Frequencies in Antiretroviral Therapy–Treated Human Immunodeficiency Virus–Infected Individuals, Clinical Infectious Diseases, Volume 66, Issue 12, 15 June 2018, Pages 1872–1882, https://doi.org/10.1093/cid/cix1116

284 Kim G, Jang MS, Son YM, Seo MJ, Ji SY, Han SH, Jung ID, Park YM, Jung HJ, Yun CH. Curcumin inhibits CD4(+) T cell activation, but augments CD69 expression and TGF-β1-mediated generation of regulatory T cells at late phase. PLoS One. 2013 Apr 26;8(4):e62300. doi: 10.1371/journal.pone.0062300. Erratum in: PLoS One. 2013;8(5). doi: 10.1371/annotation/631b0f02-bf10-4bac-88a3-c986f2b73284. PMID: 23658623; PMCID: PMC3637266.

285 Chen, J., Bruce, D. & Cantorna, M.T. Vitamin D receptor expression controls proliferation of naïve CD8+ T cells and development of CD8 mediated gastrointestinal inflammation. BMC Immunol 15, 6 (2014). https://doi.org/10.1186/1471-2172-15-6

286 Tian J, Lu Y, Zhang H, Chau CH, Dang HN, Kaufman DL. Gamma-aminobutyric acid inhibits T cell autoimmunity and the development of inflammatory responses in a mouse type 1 diabetes model. J Immunol. 2004 Oct 15;173(8):5298-304. doi: 10.4049/jimmunol.173.8.5298. PMID: 15470076.

287 Rosell, Axel et al. "Patients With COVID-19 Have Elevated Levels of Circulating Extracellular Vesicle Tissue Factor Activity That Is Associated With Severity and Mortality-Brief Report." Arteriosclerosis, thrombosis, and vascular biology vol. 41,2 (2021): 878-882. doi:10.1161/ATVBAHA.120.315547

288 Jing Wang, Theodore P. Ciaraldi, Fahumiya Samad, "Tissue Factor Expression in Obese Type 2 Diabetic Subjects and Its Regulation by Antidiabetic Agents", Journal of Obesity, vol. 2015, Article ID 291209, 8 pages, 2015. https://doi.org/10.1155/2015/291209

In the presence of Lipopolysaccharides (LPS) THC enhances TF expression
LPS is an endotoxin produced from gram-negative bacteria. Studies show that THC has a slightly deleterious effect on gram-negative bacteria [[289]].
Δ9-Tetrahydrocannabinol (THC) enhances lipopolysaccharide-stimulated tissue factor in human monocytes and monocyte-derived microvesicles[290]
Curcumin inhibits tissue factor
Inhibition of Tissue Factor Gene Activation in Cultured Endothelial Cells by Curcumin[291]
Vitamin D inhibits TF expression
Vitamin D inhibits Tissue Factor and CAMs expression in oxidized low-density lipoproteins-treated human endothelial cells by modulating NF-κB pathway.[292]
Gaba: no data found

44. FGF-2/bFGF (fiberblast growth factor/)
"Fibroblast growth factor-2 (FGF-2) is a member of a large family of proteins that bind heparin and heparan sulfate and modulate the function of a wide range of cell types. FGF-2 stimulates the growth and development of new blood vessels (angiogenesis) that contribute to the pathogenesis of several diseases (i.e. cancer, atherosclerosis), normal wound healing and tissue development."[293]
Covid-19 raises FGF2
Fibroblast Growth Factor: A Target for COVID-19 Infection[294]
Hyperglycemia raises FGF2
Hyperglycemia Mediates a Shift From Cap-Dependent to Cap-Independent Translation Via a 4E-BP1–Dependent Mechanism[295]
Cannabinoids inhibit FGF2
The FGF receptor uses the endocannabinoid signaling system to couple to an axonal growth response
Curcumin inhibits FGF2
Curcumin is an in vivo inhibitor of angiogenesis[296]
Vitamin D down-regulates FGF2
Eldecalcitol (ED-71), an analog of 1α,25(OH) 2 D 3, inhibits the growth of squamous cell carcinoma (SCC) cells in vitro and in vivo by down-regulating expression of heparin-binding protein 17/fibroblast growth factor-binding protein-1 (HBp17/FGFBP-1) and FGF-2[297]

289 Becker W, Alrafas HR, Busbee PB, Walla MD, Wilson K, Miranda K, Cai G, Putluri V, Putluri N, Nagarkatti M, Nagarkatti PS. Cannabinoid Receptor Activation on Haematopoietic Cells and Enterocytes Protects against Colitis. J Crohns Colitis. 2021 Jun 22;15(6):1032-1048. doi: 10.1093/ecco-jcc/jjaa253. PMID: 33331878; PMCID: PMC8218712

290 Williams, Julie C et al. "Δ(9)-Tetrahydrocannabinol (THC) enhances lipopolysaccharide-stimulated tissue factor in human monocytes and monocyte-derived microvesicles." Journal of inflammation (London, England) vol. 12 39. 12 Jun. 2015, doi:10.1186/s12950-015-0084-1

291 Pendurthi UR, Williams JT, Rao LV. Inhibition of tissue factor gene activation in cultured endothelial cells by curcumin. Suppression of activation of transcription factors Egr-1, AP-1, and NF-kappa B. Arterioscler Thromb Vasc Biol. 1997 Dec;17(12):3406-13. doi: 10.1161/01.atv.17.12.3406. PMID: 9437186.

292 Cimmino G, Morello A, Conte S, Pellegrino G, Marra L, Golino P, Cirillo P. Vitamin D inhibits Tissue Factor and CAMs expression in oxidized low-density lipoproteins-treated human endothelial cells by modulating NF-κB pathway. Eur J Pharmacol. 2020 Oct 15;885:173422. doi: 10.1016/j.ejphar.2020.173422. Epub 2020 Aug 2. PMID: 32755551.

293 Nugent MA, Iozzo RV. Fibroblast growth factor-2. Int J Biochem Cell Biol. 2000 Feb;32(2):115-20. doi: 10.1016/s1357-2725(99)00123-5. PMID: 10687947.

294 Cuevas, Pedro and Antonio Manquillo. "Fibroblast growth factor: A target for covid-19 infection." (2020).

295 Michael D. Dennis, Jeffrey S. Shenberger, Bruce A. Stanley, Scot R. Kimball, Leonard S. Jefferson; Hyperglycemia Mediates a Shift From Cap-Dependent to Cap-Independent Translation Via a 4E-BP1–Dependent Mechanism. Diabetes 1 July 2013; 62 (7): 2204–2214. https://doi.org/10.2337/db12-1453

296 Arbiser JL, Klauber N, Rohan R, van Leeuwen R, Huang MT, Fisher C, Flynn E, Byers HR. Curcumin is an in vivo inhibitor of angiogenesis. Mol Med. 1998 Jun;4(6):376-83. PMID: 10780880; PMCID: PMC2230271.

297 Shintani T, Takatsu F, Rosli SNZ, Usui E, Hamada A, Sumi K, Hayashido Y, Toratani S, Okamoto T. Eldecalcitol (ED-71), an analog of 1α,25(OH)2D3, inhibits the growth of squamous cell carcinoma (SCC) cells in vitro and in vivo by down-regulating expression of heparin-binding protein 17/fibroblast growth factor-binding protein-1 (HBp17/FGFBP-1) and FGF-2. In Vitro Cell Dev Biol Anim. 2017 Oct;53(9):810-817. doi: 10.1007/s11626-017-0183-9. Epub 2017 Jul 14. PMID:

Gaba: no data found

45. PDGF (platelet-derived growth factor)

"Platelet-derived growth factor (PDGF) constitutes a family of dimeric isoforms, acting on connective tissue cells and certain other cell types. PDGF was originally discovered as a constituent of platelets, which are released into serum in conjunction with blood coagulation. Although the α-granules of platelets are a major storage site for PDGF, PDGF is also produced by many other cell types. PDGF stimulates the growth of its target cells, but also affects chemotaxis, i.e., directed cell movement, and cell shape through reorganization of the actin filament system. PDGF also affects the differentiation of specific cell types and promotes cell survival. Through these effects, PDGF has important functions in certain organs during embryonic development, as well as in the adult in the stimulation of wound healing and in the maintenance of connective tissue homeostasis. Overactivity of PDGF has been linked to certain diseases, such as malignancies in which PDGF production may promote tumor growth via autocrine or paracrine stimulation. PDGF is also implicated in other disorders that involve an excess of cell proliferation, e.g., atherosclerosis and fibrotic conditions."[298]

Covid-19 raises PDGF

Pulmonary Procoagulant and Innate Immune Responses in Critically Ill COVID-19 Patients[299]

PDGF regulates Glucose transporter expression

Platelet-derived growth factor regulates glucose transporter expression[300]

Cannabinoids inhibit PDGF

Repurposing Cannabidiol as a Potential Drug Candidate for Anti-Tumor Therapies[301]

Curcumin inhibits PDGF

Curcumin inhibits platelet-derived growth factor-stimulated vascular smooth muscle cell function and injury-induced neointima formation[302]

Lower levels of Vitamin D correlate with higher levels of PDGF

The Role of Vitamin D, Platelet-Derived Growth Factor and Insulin-Like Growth Factor 1 in the Progression of Thyroid Diseases[303]

PDGF inhibits Gaba receptors

Platelet-derived growth factor receptor is a novel modulator of type A gamma-aminobutyric acid-gated ion channels[304]

28710602.

298 Carl-Henrik Heldin, in Encyclopedia of Hormones, 2003

299 Nossent, Esther J et al. "Pulmonary Procoagulant and Innate Immune Responses in Critically Ill COVID-19 Patients." Frontiers in immunology vol. 12 664209. 14 May. 2021, doi:10.3389/fimmu.2021.664209

300 Rollins BJ, Morrison ED, Usher P, Flier JS. Platelet-derived growth factor regulates glucose transporter expression. J Biol Chem. 1988 Nov 15;263(32):16523-6. PMID: 3182801.

301 Wang F, Multhoff G. Repurposing Cannabidiol as a Potential Drug Candidate for Anti-Tumor Therapies. Biomolecules. 2021 Apr 15;11(4):582. doi: 10.3390/biom11040582. PMID: 33921049; PMCID: PMC8071421.

302 Yang X, Thomas DP, Zhang X, Culver BW, Alexander BM, Murdoch WJ, Rao MN, Tulis DA, Ren J, Sreejayan N. Curcumin inhibits platelet-derived growth factor-stimulated vascular smooth muscle cell function and injury-induced neointima formation. Arterioscler Thromb Vasc Biol. 2006 Jan;26(1):85-90. doi: 10.1161/01.ATV.0000191635.00744.b6. Epub 2005 Oct 20. PMID: 16239599.

303 Abdellateif, Mona S et al. "The Role of Vitamin D, Platelet-Derived Growth Factor and Insulin-Like Growth Factor 1 in the Progression of Thyroid Diseases." Asian Pacific journal of cancer prevention : APJCP vol. 21,7 2083-2089. 1 Jul. 2020, doi:10.31557/APJCP.2020.21.7.2083

304 Valenzuela CF, Kazlauskas A, Brozowski SJ, Weiner JL, Demali KA, McDonald BJ, Moss SJ, Dunwiddie TV, Harris RA. Platelet-derived growth factor receptor is a novel modulator of type A gamma-aminobutyric acid-gated ion channels. Mol Pharmacol. 1995 Dec;48(6):1099-107. PMID: 8848010.

Protein coding gene

46. C1q (C1 complex)

"C1q is the first subcomponent of the C1 complex of the classical pathway of complement activation. Several functions have been assigned to C1q, which include antibody-dependent and independent immune functions, and are considered to be mediated by C1q receptors present on the effector cell surface. There remains some uncertainty about the identities of the receptors that mediate C1q functions. [305]." (*C1q: structure, function, and receptors*)

Covid-19 decreases C1q
Clinical Characteristics and Immune Injury Mechanisms in 71 Patients with COVID-19 [306]

C1q regulates glucose
O-GlcNAc Transferase/Host Cell Factor C1 Complex Regulates Gluconeogenesis by Modulating PGC-1α Stability [307]

Cannabinoids upregulate C1q
Cannabidiol Improves Cognitive Impairment and Reverses Cortical Transcriptional Changes Induced by Ketamine, in Schizophrenia-Like Model in Rats[308]
Curcumin: no data found

Vitamin D deficiency reduces C1q
Vitamin D deficiency as marker for disease activity and damage in systemic lupus erythematosus: a comparison with anti-dsDNA and anti-C1q[309]
Gaba: no data found

Substances Related to Cognitive Decline

47. Phosphorylated Tau

"Tau is a microtubule-stabilizing protein that plays an important role in the formation of axonal microtubules in neurons. Phosphorylated tau (p-Tau) has received great attention in the field of Alzheimer's disease (AD) as a potential therapeutic target due to its involvement with synaptic damage and neuronal dysfunction. Mounting evidence suggests that amyloid beta (Aβ)-targeted clinical trials continuously failed; therefore, it is important to consider alternative therapeutic strategies such as p-tau-PROTACs targeted small molecules for AD and other tauopathies." (Phosphorylated tau targeted small-molecule PROTACs for the treatment of Alzheimer's disease and tauopathies[310])

305 Kishore U, Reid KB. C1q: structure, function, and receptors. Immunopharmacology. 2000 Aug;49(1-2):159-70. doi: 10.1016/s0162-3109(00)80301-x. PMID: 10904115.

306 Wu Y, Huang X, Sun J, Xie T, Lei Y, Muhammad J, Li X, Zeng X, Zhou F, Qin H, Shao L, Zhang Q. Clinical Characteristics and Immune Injury Mechanisms in 71 Patients with COVID-19. mSphere. 2020 Jul 15;5(4):e00362-20. doi: 10.1128/mSphere.00362-20. PMID: 32669467; PMCID: PMC7364211.

307 Ruan HB, Han X, Li MD, Singh JP, Qian K, Azarhoush S, Zhao L, Bennett AM, Samuel VT, Wu J, Yates JR 3rd, Yang X. O-GlcNAc transferase/host cell factor C1 complex regulates gluconeogenesis by modulating PGC-1α stability. Cell Metab. 2012 Aug 8;16(2):226-37. doi: 10.1016/j.cmet.2012.07.006. PMID: 22883232; PMCID: PMC3480732.

308 Kozela E, Krawczyk M, Kos T, Juknat A, Vogel Z, Popik P. Cannabidiol Improves Cognitive Impairment and Reverses Cortical Transcriptional Changes Induced by Ketamine, in Schizophrenia-Like Model in Rats. Mol Neurobiol. 2020 Mar;57(3):1733-1747. doi: 10.1007/s12035-019-01831-2. Epub 2019 Dec 11. PMID: 31823199.

309 Mok CC, Birmingham DJ, Ho LY, Hebert LA, Song H, Rovin BH. Vitamin D deficiency as marker for disease activity and damage in systemic lupus erythematosus: a comparison with anti-dsDNA and anti-C1q. Lupus. 2012 Jan;21(1):36-42. doi: 10.1177/0961203311422094. Epub 2011 Oct 12. PMID: 21993384.

310 Jangampalli Adi P, Reddy PH. Phosphorylated tau targeted small-molecule PROTACs for the treatment of Alzheimer's disease and tauopathies. Biochim Biophys Acta Mol Basis Dis. 2021 Aug 1;1867(8):166162. doi: 10.1016/j.bbadis.2021.166162. Epub 2021 Apr 30. PMID: 33940164; PMCID: PMC8154736.

Phosphorylated Tau is raised in Covid-19
Alzheimer's-like signaling in brains of COVID-19 patients[311]
High Glucose forms phosporylated Tau
High glucose induces formation of tau hyperphosphorylation via Cav-1-mTOR pathway: A potential molecular mechanism for diabetes-induced cognitive dysfunction[312]
Cannabinoids reduce phosphorylated Tau
Cannabinoids for treatment of Alzheimer's disease: moving toward the clinic[313]
Curcumin decreases hyperphosphorylation of Tau
Curcumin Decreases Hyperphosphorylation of Tau by Down-Regulating Caveolin-1/GSK-3β in N2a/APP695swe Cells and APP/PS1 Double Transgenic Alzheimer's Disease Mice[314]
Vitamin D inhibits Tau
Activation of vitamin D receptor inhibits Tau phosphorylation is associated with reduction of iron accumulation in APP/PS1 transgenic mice[315]
Gaba reduces Tau binding
γ-Aminobutyric acid type A (GABA) receptor activation modulates tau phosphorylation[316]

48. AB (B-Amyloid)

"The amyloid β peptide (Aβ) is a critical initiator that triggers the progression of Alzheimer's Disease (AD) via accumulation and aggregation, of which the process may be caused by Aβ overproduction or perturbation clearance. Aβ is generated from amyloid precursor protein through sequential cleavage of β- and γ-secretases while Aβ removal is dependent on the proteolysis and lysosome degradation system." (β-Amyloid: the key peptide in the pathogenesis of Alzheimer's disease[317])

Covid-19 raises b-amyloid
B-Amyloid Deposits in Young COVID Patients (preprint)[318]
High Glucose elevates amyloid
High glucose induces formation of tau hyperphosphorylation via Cav-1-mTOR pathway: A potential molecular mechanism for diabetes-induced cognitive dysfunction[319]

311 Reiken, Steven & Sittenfeld, Leah & Dridi, Haikel & Liu, Yang & Liu, Xiaoping & Marks, Andrew. (2022). Alzheimer's-like signaling in brains of COVID-19 patients. Alzheimer's & Dementia. 10.1002/alz.12558.

312 Wu, Jing et al. "High glucose induces formation of tau hyperphosphorylation via Cav-1-mTOR pathway: A potential molecular mechanism for diabetes-induced cognitive dysfunction." Oncotarget vol. 8,25 (2017): 40843-40856. doi:10.18632/oncotarget.17257

313 Aso E, Ferrer I. Cannabinoids for treatment of Alzheimer's disease: moving toward the clinic. Front Pharmacol. 2014 Mar 5;5:37. doi: 10.3389/fphar.2014.00037. PMID: 24634659; PMCID: PMC3942876.

314 Sun J, Zhang X, Wang C, Teng Z, Li Y. Curcumin Decreases Hyperphosphorylation of Tau by Down-Regulating Caveolin-1/GSK-3β in N2a/APP695swe Cells and APP/PS1 Double Transgenic Alzheimer's Disease Mice. Am J Chin Med. 2017;45(8):1667-1682. doi: 10.1142/S0192415X17500902. Epub 2017 Nov 13. PMID: 29132216.

315 Wu TY, Zhao LX, Zhang YH, Fan YG. Activation of vitamin D receptor inhibits Tau phosphorylation is associated with reduction of iron accumulation in APP/PS1 transgenic mice. Neurochem Int. 2022 Feb;153:105260. doi: 10.1016/j.neuint.2021.105260. Epub 2021 Dec 22. PMID: 34953963.

316 Nykänen NP, Kysenius K, Sakha P, Tammela P, Huttunen HJ. γ-Aminobutyric acid type A (GABAA) receptor activation modulates tau phosphorylation. J Biol Chem. 2012 Feb 24;287(9):6743-52. doi: 10.1074/jbc.M111.309385. Epub 2012 Jan 10. PMID: 22235112; PMCID: PMC3307276.

317 Sun X, Chen WD, Wang YD. β-Amyloid: the key peptide in the pathogenesis of Alzheimer's disease. Front Pharmacol. 2015 Sep 30;6:221. doi: 10.3389/fphar.2015.00221. PMID: 26483691; PMCID: PMC4588032.

318 Rhodes, C. Harker and Priemer, David S. and Karlovich, Esma and Perl, Daniel P. and Goldman, James, B-Amyloid Deposits in Young COVID Patients. Available at SSRN: https://ssrn.com/abstract=4003213 or http://dx.doi.org/10.2139/ssrn.4003213

319 Matthew K Taylor, Debra K Sullivan, Russell H Swerdlow, Eric D Vidoni, Jill K Morris, Jonathan D Mahnken, Jeffrey M Burns, A high-glycemic diet is associated with cerebral amyloid burden in cognitively normal older adults, The American Journal of Clinical Nutrition, Volume 106, Issue 6, December 2017, Pages 1463–1470, https://doi.org/10.3945/ajcn.117.162263

Cannabinoids reduce b-amyloid
Amyloid proteotoxicity initiates an inflammatory response blocked by cannabinoids[320]
Curcumin inhibits formation of b-amyloid
Curcumin Inhibits Formation of Amyloid β Oligomers and Fibrils, Binds Plaques, and Reduces Amyloid in Vivo[321]
Vitamin D helps clear b-amyloid
Genomic and Nongenomic Signaling Induced by 1α,25(OH)2-Vitamin D3 Promotes the Recovery of Amyloid-β Phagocytosis by Alzheimer's Disease Macrophages[322]
Gaba down-regulates b-amyloid
GABA attenuates amyloid toxicity by downregulating its endocytosis and improves cognitive impairment[323]

49. CCL11 (Eotaxin-1)

"CCL11 was discovered as a result of a systematic search for eosinophil chemotactic factors in bronchoalveolar lavage fluid in a guinea pig asthma model. Despite the relatively low level of sequence identity among the "eotaxins" (34–38%), they all bind to the receptor CCR3, which is expressed at high levels on eosinophils and basophils."[324]

Covid-19 raises CCL11 (Eotaxin-1)
Eotaxin-1 (CCL11) in neuroinflammatory disorders and possible role in COVID-19 neurologic complications[325]

High levels of CCL11 (Eotaxin-1) are linked to Diabetes
Orally administered anti-eotaxin-1 monoclonal antibody is biologically active in the gut and alleviates immune-mediated hepatitis: A novel anti-inflammatory personalized therapeutic approach[326]

Cannabinoid THC Increases CCL11 (Eotaxin-1)*
Cannabis use is associated with increased CCL11 plasma levels in young healthy volunteers[327]
*See **Considerations**.
Cannabinoid CBD decreases CCL11 (Eotaxin-1)
In Vitro Effects of Cannabidiol on Activated Immune-Inflammatory Pathways in Major Depressive Patients and Healthy Controls[328]

320 Currais, A., Quehenberger, O., M Armando, A. et al. Amyloid proteotoxicity initiates an inflammatory response blocked by cannabinoids. npj Aging Mech Dis 2, 16012 (2016). https://doi.org/10.1038/npjamd.2016.12
321 Yang F, Lim GP, Begum AN, Ubeda OJ, Simmons MR, Ambegaokar SS, Chen PP, Kayed R, Glabe CG, Frautschy SA, Cole GM. Curcumin inhibits formation of amyloid beta oligomers and fibrils, binds plaques, and reduces amyloid in vivo. J Biol Chem. 2005 Feb 18;280(7):5892-901. doi: 10.1074/jbc.M404751200. Epub 2004 Dec 7. PMID: 15590663.
322 Mizwicki MT, Menegaz D, Zhang J, Barrientos-Durán A, Tse S, Cashman JR, Griffin PR, Fiala M. Genomic and nongenomic signaling induced by 1α,25(OH)2-vitamin D3 promotes the recovery of amyloid-β phagocytosis by Alzheimer's disease macrophages. J Alzheimers Dis. 2012;29(1):51-62. doi: 10.3233/JAD-2012-110560. PMID: 22207005.
323 Sun X, Meng X, Zhang J, Li Y, Wang L, Qin X, Sui N, Zhang Y. GABA attenuates amyloid toxicity by downregulating its endocytosis and improves cognitive impairment. J Alzheimers Dis. 2012;31(3):635-49. doi: 10.3233/JAD-2012-120535. PMID: 22672879.
324 Ronald L. Rabin, in Encyclopedia of Hormones, 2003
325 Nazarinia D, Behzadifard M, Gholampour J, Karimi R, Gholampour M. Eotaxin-1 (CCL11) in neuroinflammatory disorders and possible role in COVID-19 neurologic complications. Acta Neurol Belg. 2022 Aug;122(4):865-869. doi: 10.1007/s13760-022-01984-3. Epub 2022 Jun 12. PMID: 35690992; PMCID: PMC9188656.
326 Khoury T, Rotnemer-Golinkin D, Zolotarev L, Ilan Y. Orally administered anti-eotaxin-1 monoclonal antibody is biologically active in the gut and alleviates immune-mediated hepatitis: A novel anti-inflammatory personalized therapeutic approach. Int J Immunopathol Pharmacol. 2021 Jan-Dec;35:20587384211021215. doi: 10.1177/20587384211021215. PMID: 34275345; PMCID: PMC8287423.
327 Fernandez-Egea E, Scoriels L, Theegala S, Giro M, Ozanne SE, Burling K, Jones PB. Cannabis use is associated with increased CCL11 plasma levels in young healthy volunteers. Prog Neuropsychopharmacol Biol Psychiatry. 2013 Oct 1;46:25-8. doi: 10.1016/j.pnpbp.2013.06.011. Epub 2013 Jun 29. PMID: 23820464.

Curcumin decreases CCL11 (Eotaxin-1)
Involvement of p38 MAPK, JNK, p42/p44 ERK and NF-κB in IL-1β-induced chemokine release in human airway smooth muscle cells[329]
Vitamin D decreases CCL11 (Eotaxin-1)
Vitamin D decreases the secretion of eotaxin and RANTES in nasal polyp fibroblasts derived from Taiwanese patients with chronic rhinosinusitis with nasal polyps[330]
Gaba: No data

Substances related to bronchoconstriction

50. CD147/BSG/EMMPRIN (Basigin/extracellular matrix metalloproteinase inducer/cluster of differentiation 147)

"CD147, a transmembrane glycoprotein, is expressed on all leukocytes, platelets, and endothelial cells. It has been implicated in a variety of physiological and pathological activities through interacting with multiple partners, including cyclophilins, monocarboxylate transporters, Caveolin-1, and integrins. While CD147 is best known as a potent inducer of extracellular matrix metalloproteinases (hence also called EMMPRIN), it can also function as a key mediator of inflammatory and immune responses. Increased expression of CD147 has been implicated in the pathogenesis of a number of diseases, such as asthma-mediated lung inflammation, rheumatoid arthritis, multiple sclerosis, myocardial infarction and ischemic stroke." (*CD147: a novel modulator of inflammatory and immune disorders*[331])

Covid-19 raises CD147
Distribution of ACE2, CD147, CD26, and other SARS-CoV-2 associated molecules in tissues and immune cells in health and in asthma, COPD, obesity, hypertension, and COVID-19 risk factors[332]

High Glucose raises CD147
Distribution of ACE2, CD147, CD26, and other SARS-CoV-2 associated molecules in tissues and immune cells in health and in asthma, COPD, obesity, hypertension, and COVID-19 risk factors[333]

Cannabinoids lower expression of CD147
Anti-Cancer Potential of Cannabinoids, Terpenes, and Flavonoids Present in Cannabis[334]

---

328 Rachayon M, Jirakran K, Sodsai P, Klinchanhom S, Sughondhabirom A, Plaimas K, Suratanee A, Maes M. In Vitro Effects of Cannabidiol on Activated Immune-Inflammatory Pathways in Major Depressive Patients and Healthy Controls. Pharmaceuticals (Basel). 2022 Mar 26;15(4):405. doi: 10.3390/ph15040405. PMID: 35455402; PMCID: PMC9032852.

329 Wuyts WA, Vanaudenaerde BM, Dupont LJ, Demedts MG, Verleden GM. Involvement of p38 MAPK, JNK, p42/p44 ERK and NF-kappaB in IL-1beta-induced chemokine release in human airway smooth muscle cells. Respir Med. 2003 Jul;97(7):811-7. doi: 10.1016/s0954-6111(03)00036-2. PMID: 12854631.

330 Wang LF, Chien CY, Tai CF, Chiang FY, Chen JY. Vitamin D decreases the secretion of eotaxin and RANTES in nasal polyp fibroblasts derived from Taiwanese patients with chronic rhinosinusitis with nasal polyps. Kaohsiung J Med Sci. 2015 Feb;31(2):63-9. doi: 10.1016/j.kjms.2014.11.011. Epub 2014 Dec 17. PMID: 25645983.

331 Zhu X, Song Z, Zhang S, Nanda A, Li G. CD147: a novel modulator of inflammatory and immune disorders. Curr Med Chem. 2014;21(19):2138-45. doi: 10.2174/0929867321666131227163352. PMID: 24372217.

332 Radzikowska U, Ding M, Tan G, Zhakparov D, Peng Y, Wawrzyniak P, Wang M, Li S, Morita H, Altunbulakli C, Reiger M, Neumann AU, Lunjani N, Traidl-Hoffmann C, Nadeau KC, O'Mahony L, Akdis C, Sokolowska M. Distribution of ACE2, CD147, CD26, and other SARS-CoV-2 associated molecules in tissues and immune cells in health and in asthma, COPD, obesity, hypertension, and COVID-19 risk factors. Allergy. 2020 Nov;75(11):2829-2845. doi: 10.1111/all.14429. Epub 2020 Aug 24. PMID: 32496587; PMCID: PMC7300910.

333 Radzikowska U, Ding M, Tan G, Zhakparov D, Peng Y, Wawrzyniak P, Wang M, Li S, Morita H, Altunbulakli C, Reiger M, Neumann AU, Lunjani N, Traidl-Hoffmann C, Nadeau KC, O'Mahony L, Akdis C, Sokolowska M. Distribution of ACE2, CD147, CD26, and other SARS-CoV-2 associated molecules in tissues and immune cells in health and in asthma, COPD, obesity, hypertension, and COVID-19 risk factors. Allergy. 2020 Nov;75(11):2829-2845. doi: 10.1111/all.14429. Epub 2020 Aug 24. PMID: 32496587; PMCID: PMC7300910.

Curcumin inhibits CD147
Curcumin inhibits EMMPRIN and MMP-9 expression through AMPK-MAPK and PKC signaling in PMA induced macrophages[335]
Vitamin D: no data found
Gaba: no data found

51. LTB4 (Leukotriene b4)
"Leukotriene B4 and the cys-LTs were increased in exhaled breath condensate from asthmatic subjects compared with healthy controls.188 After allergen challenge, there was a significant increase in leukotriene levels in the BAL fluid of allergic subjects, and this was associated with increased eosinophilic inflammation and bronchial responsiveness.189 Leukotriene levels in induced sputum from asthmatic subjects exceed those found in nonasthmatic controls and correlate with severity of disease."[336]

Leukotrines are raised in Covid-19
The Leukotriene Receptor Antagonist Montelukast as a Potential COVID-19 Therapeutic[337]

Leukotrines impact insulin receptor signaling
Leukotriene Involvement in the Insulin Receptor Pathway and Macrophage Profiles in Muscles from Type 1 Diabetic Mice[338]

Cannabinoids decrease LTB4
5-Lipoxygenase and anandamide hydrolase (FAAH) mediate the antitumor activity of cannabidiol, a non-psychoactive cannabinoid[339]
Effect of endocannabinoids on IgE-mediated allergic response in RBL-2H3 cells[340]

Curcumin inhibits LTB4
Curcumin: a potent inhibitor of leukotriene B4 formation in rat peritoneal polymorphonuclear neutrophils (PMNL)[341]

Vitamin D decreases LTB4
5-Lipoxygenase (ALOX5): Genetic susceptibility to type 2 diabetes and vitamin D effects on monocytes[342]

Gaba: no data found

334 Tomko AM, Whynot EG, Ellis LD, Dupré DJ. Anti-Cancer Potential of Cannabinoids, Terpenes, and Flavonoids Present in Cannabis. Cancers. 2020; 12(7):1985. https://doi.org/10.3390/cancers12071985

335 Cao J, Han Z, Tian L, Chen K, Fan Y, Ye B, Huang W, Wang C, Huang Z. Curcumin inhibits EMMPRIN and MMP-9 expression through AMPK-MAPK and PKC signaling in PMA induced macrophages. J Transl Med. 2014 Sep 21;12:266. doi: 10.1186/s12967-014-0266-2. PMID: 25241044; PMCID: PMC4205290.

336 A. Wesley Burks MD, in Middleton's Allergy: Principles and Practice, 2020

337 Aigner L, Pietrantonio F, Bessa de Sousa DM, Michael J, Schuster D, Reitsamer HA, Zerbe H, Studnicka M. The Leukotriene Receptor Antagonist Montelukast as a Potential COVID-19 Therapeutic. Front Mol Biosci. 2020 Dec 17;7:610132. doi: 10.3389/fmolb.2020.610132. PMID: 33392263; PMCID: PMC7773944.

338 João Pedro Tôrres Guimarães, Luciano Ribeiro Filgueiras, Joilson Oliveira Martins, Sonia Jancar, "Leukotriene Involvement in the Insulin Receptor Pathway and Macrophage Profiles in Muscles from Type 1 Diabetic Mice", Mediators of Inflammation, vol. 2019, Article ID 4596127, 8 pages, 2019. https://doi.org/10.1155/2019/4596127

339 Massi P, Valenti M, Vaccani A, Gasperi V, Perletti G, Marras E, Fezza F, Maccarrone M, Parolaro D. 5-Lipoxygenase and anandamide hydrolase (FAAH) mediate the antitumor activity of cannabidiol, a non-psychoactive cannabinoid. J Neurochem. 2008 Feb;104(4):1091-100. doi: 10.1111/j.1471-4159.2007.05073.x. Epub 2007 Nov 17. PMID: 18028339.

340 Yoo JM, Sok DE, Kim MR. Effect of endocannabinoids on IgE-mediated allergic response in RBL-2H3 cells. Int Immunopharmacol. 2013 Sep;17(1):123-31. doi: 10.1016/j.intimp.2013.05.013. Epub 2013 Jun 1. PMID: 23731947.

341 Ammon HP, Anazodo MI, Safayhi H, Dhawan BN, Srimal RC. Curcumin: a potent inhibitor of leukotriene B4 formation in rat peritoneal polymorphonuclear neutrophils (PMNL). Planta Med. 1992 Apr;58(2):226. doi: 10.1055/s-2006-961438. Erratum in: Planta Med 1993 Feb;59(1):100. PMID: 1326775.

342 Nejatian N, Häfner AK, Shoghi F, Badenhoop K, Penna-Martinez M. 5-Lipoxygenase (ALOX5): Genetic susceptibility to type 2 diabetes and vitamin D effects on monocytes. J Steroid Biochem Mol Biol. 2019 Mar;187:52-57. doi: 10.1016/j.jsbmb.2018.10.022. Epub 2018 Dec 3. PMID: 30521849.

Detoxification

52. EPHX1 (Epoxide hydrolase 1/Microsomal epoxide hydrolase)
"epoxide hydrolase is a critical biotransformation enzyme that converts epoxides from the degradation of aromatic compounds to trans-dihydrodiols which can be conjugated and excreted from the body. Epoxide hydrolase functions in both the activation and detoxification of epoxides. Mutations in this gene cause preeclampsia, epoxide hydrolase deficiency or increased epoxide hydrolase activity. Alternatively spliced transcript variants encoding the same protein have been found for this gene. [provided by RefSeq, Dec 2008]" (*EPHX1 Epoxide hydrolase 1, National Library of Medicine, NIH*)

Increasing epoxy fatty acids (EET, EEQ, and EDP) by inhibiting EPHX1 could treat Covid-19
Activating endogenous resolution pathways by soluble epoxide hydrolase inhibitors for the management of COVID-19[343]

Inhibiting EPHX1 lowers blood sugar
Inhibition or Deletion of Soluble Epoxide Hydrolase Prevents Hyperglycemia, Promotes Insulin Secretion, and Reduces Islet Apoptosis[344]

Cannabinoid (CBD) boosts EPHX1
Pathways and gene networks mediating the regulatory effects of cannabidiol, a nonpsychoactive cannabinoid, in autoimmune T cells

Curcumin up-regulates EPHX1, then down-regulates after 48 hours
Time- and dose-dependent effects of curcumin on gene expression in human colon cancer cells[345]

Vitamin D decreases EPHX1
Vitamin D, DNA methylation, and breast cancer[346]
Gaba: no data found

Immune response

53. FOXP3 (scurfin, forkhead box P3)
"FOXP3 is a member of the forkhead transcription factor family. Unlike other members, it is mainly expressed in a subset of CD4+ T-cells that play a suppressive role in the immune system. A function of FOXP3 is to suppress the function of NFAT and NFkappaB and this leads to suppression ofexpression of many genes including IL-2 and effector T-cell cytokines." (*FOXP3 and its role in the immune system*[347])

Severe Covid-19 lowers FOXP3
Upregulation of FOXP3 is associated with severity of hypoxia and poor outcomes in COVID-19 patients[348]

---

343 Manickam M, Meenakshisundaram S, Pillaiyar T. Activating endogenous resolution pathways by soluble epoxide hydrolase inhibitors for the management of COVID-19. Arch Pharm (Weinheim). 2022 Mar;355(3):e2100367. doi: 10.1002/ardp.202100367. Epub 2021 Nov 21. PMID: 34802171; PMCID: PMC9011438.

344 Luo P, Chang HH, Zhou Y, Zhang S, Hwang SH, Morisseau C, Wang CY, Inscho EW, Hammock BD, Wang MH. Inhibition or deletion of soluble epoxide hydrolase prevents hyperglycemia, promotes insulin secretion, and reduces islet apoptosis. J Pharmacol Exp Ther. 2010 Aug;334(2):430-8. doi: 10.1124/jpet.110.167544. Epub 2010 May 3. PMID: 20439437; PMCID: PMC2913776.

345 Van Erk, Marjan J et al. "Time- and dose-dependent effects of curcumin on gene expression in human colon cancer cells." Journal of carcinogenesis vol. 3,1 8. 12 May. 2004, doi:10.1186/1477-3163-3-8

346 O'Brien, K.M., Sandler, D.P., Xu, Z. et al. Vitamin D, DNA methylation, and breast cancer. Breast Cancer Res 20, 70 (2018). https://doi.org/10.1186/s13058-018-0994-y

347 Kim CH. FOXP3 and its role in the immune system. Adv Exp Med Biol. 2009;665:17-29. doi: 10.1007/978-1-4419-1599-3_2. PMID: 20429413.

Obesity lowers FOXP3
Type 2 Diabetes: How Much of an Autoimmune Disease?[349]
Cannabinoids increase FOXP3
Cannabidiol (CBD) Induces Functional Tregs in Response to Low-Level T Cell Activation[350]
Curcumin increases FOXP3
Curcumin regulates the differentiation of naïve CD4+T cells and activates IL-10 immune modulation against acute lung injury in mice[351]
Vitamin D promotes FOXP3 expression
1,25(OH)2 vitamin D3 promotes FOXP3 expression via binding to vitamin D response elements in its conserved non-coding sequence region[352]
Gaba: no data found

54. NLRP3 (NLR family pyrin domain containing 3)

"The NLRP3 inflammasome is a critical component of the innate immune system that mediates caspase-1 activation and the secretion of proinflammatory cytokines IL-1β/IL-18 in response to microbial infection and cellular damage. However, the aberrant activation of the NLRP3 inflammasome has been linked with several inflammatory disorders, which include cryopyrin-associated periodic syndromes, Alzheimer's disease, diabetes, and atherosclerosis. The NLRP3 inflammasome is activated by diverse stimuli, and multiple molecular and cellular events, including ionic flux, mitochondrial dysfunction, and the production of reactive oxygen species, and lysosomal damage have been shown to trigger its activation. How NLRP3 responds to those signaling events and initiates the assembly of the NLRP3 inflammasome is not fully understood." (The NLRP3 Inflammasome: An Overview of Mechanisms of Activation and Regulation[353])
Nutraceutical Strategies for Suppressing NLRP3 Inflammasome Activation: Pertinence to the Management of COVID-19 and Beyond
Covid-19 activates NLRP3
Targeting the NLRP3 Inflammasome in Severe COVID-19[354]
High Glucose could activate NLRP3
NLRP3 Inflammasome as a Molecular Marker in Diabetic Cardiomyopathy[355]

---

348 Abdelhafiz, Ahmed S et al. "Upregulation of FOXP3 is associated with severity of hypoxia and poor outcomes in COVID-19 patients." Virology vol. 563 (2021): 74-81. doi:10.1016/j.virol.2021.08.012

349 Authors: Candia Paola, Prattichizzo Francesco, Garavelli Silvia, De Rosa Veronica, Galgani Mario, Di Rella Francesca, Spagnuolo Maria Immacolata, Colamatteo Alessandra, Fusco Clorinda, Micillo Teresa, Bruzzaniti Sara, Ceriello Antonio, Puca Annibale A., Matarese Giuseppe. Type 2 Diabetes: How Much of an Autoimmune Disease? Frontiers in Endocrinology. Volume 10, 2019. https://www.frontiersin.org/article/10.3389/fendo.2019.00451 DOI=10.3389/fendo.2019.00451 ISSN=1664-2392

350 Dhital, Saphala et al. "Cannabidiol (CBD) induces functional Tregs in response to low-level T cell activation." Cellular immunology vol. 312 (2017): 25-34. doi:10.1016/j.cellimm.2016.11.006

351 Chai YS, Chen YQ, Lin SH, Xie K, Wang CJ, Yang YZ, Xu F. Curcumin regulates the differentiation of naïve CD4+T cells and activates IL-10 immune modulation against acute lung injury in mice. Biomed Pharmacother. 2020 May;125:109946. doi: 10.1016/j.biopha.2020.109946. Epub 2020 Jan 28. PMID: 32004976.

352 Kang, Seong Wook et al. "1,25-Dihyroxyvitamin D3 promotes FOXP3 expression via binding to vitamin D response elements in its conserved noncoding sequence region." Journal of immunology (Baltimore, Md. : 1950) vol. 188,11 (2012): 5276-82. doi:10.4049/jimmunol.1101211

353 Kelley N, Jeltema D, Duan Y, He Y. The NLRP3 Inflammasome: An Overview of Mechanisms of Activation and Regulation. Int J Mol Sci. 2019 Jul 6;20(13):3328. doi: 10.3390/ijms20133328. PMID: 31284572; PMCID: PMC6651423.

354 Freeman TL, Swartz TH. Targeting the NLRP3 Inflammasome in Severe COVID-19. Front Immunol. 2020 Jun 23;11:1518. doi: 10.3389/fimmu.2020.01518. PMID: 32655582; PMCID: PMC7324760.

355 Luo, Beibei et al. "NLRP3 Inflammasome as a Molecular Marker in Diabetic Cardiomyopathy." Frontiers in physiology vol. 8 519. 25 Jul. 2017, doi:10.3389/fphys.2017.00519

Cannabinoids reduce NLRP3
Cannabidiol Modulates the Immunophenotype and Inhibits the Activation of the Inflammasome in Human Gingival Mesenchymal Stem Cells[356]
Curcumin inhibits NLRP3
Curcumin Reduces Neuronal Loss and Inhibits the NLRP3 Inflammasome Activation in an Epileptic Rat Model[357]
Vitamin D inhibits NLRP3
1,25(OH)2D3 alleviates DSS-induced ulcerative colitis via inhibiting NLRP3 inflammasome activation[358]
Gaba inhibits NLRP3
<u>*GABA transporter sustains IL-1β production in macrophages[359]*</u>

Discussion

An overactive immune system triggers the "cytokine storm," the cause of the COVID-19 pneumonia [360]. For this reason, selective immune-modulators, and immune-suppressants are needed, to counter this effect. A list of natural immunosuppressant agents has been proposed, with curcumin as one of them. This proposal include substances that have only been found to improve only half a dozen of these biomarkers. The curcumin citations are far less than in this document [361]. Prescription drugs used for immune-suppression can have severe side effects [362]. However, all four supplements have been found to have selective immune-suppressant properties, and should no

356 Libro, Rosaliana et al. "Cannabidiol Modulates the Immunophenotype and Inhibits the Activation of the Inflammasome in Human Gingival Mesenchymal Stem Cells." Frontiers in physiology vol. 7 559. 24 Nov. 2016, doi:10.3389/fphys.2016.00559

357 He Q, Jiang L, Man S, Wu L, Hu Y, Chen W. Curcumin Reduces Neuronal Loss and Inhibits the NLRP3 Inflammasome Activation in an Epileptic Rat Model. Curr Neurovasc Res. 2018;15(3):186-192. doi: 10.2174/1567202615666180731100224. PMID: 30062967; PMCID: PMC6327116.

358 Cao R, Ma Y, Li S, Shen D, Yang S, Wang X, Cao Y, Wang Z, Wei Y, Li S, Liu G, Zhang H, Wang Y, Ma Y. 1,25(OH)2 D3 alleviates DSS-induced ulcerative colitis via inhibiting NLRP3 inflammasome activation. J Leukoc Biol. 2020 Jul;108(1):283-295. doi: 10.1002/JLB.3MA0320-406RR. Epub 2020 Apr 1. PMID: 32237257.

359 Xia Y, He F, Wu X, Tan B, Chen S, Liao Y, Qi M, Chen S, Peng Y, Yin Y, Ren W. GABA transporter sustains IL-1β production in macrophages. Sci Adv. 2021 Apr 7;7(15):eabe9274. doi: 10.1126/sciadv.abe9274. PMID: 33827820; PMCID: PMC8026138.

360 Napoli C, Benincasa G, Criscuolo C, Faenza M, Liberato C, Rusciano M. Immune reactivity during COVID-19: Implications for treatment. Immunol Lett. 2021 Mar;231:28-34. doi: 10.1016/j.imlet.2021.01.001. Epub 2021 Jan 6. PMID: 33421440; PMCID: PMC7787505.

361 Peter AE, Sandeep BV, Rao BG, Kalpana VL. Calming the Storm: Natural Immunosuppressants as Adjuvants to Target the Cytokine Storm in COVID-19. Front Pharmacol. 2021 Jan 27;11:583777. doi: 10.3389/fphar.2020.583777. PMID: 33708109; PMCID: PMC7941276.

362 Cockburn N, Pateman K, Taing MW, Pradhan A, Ford PJ. Managing the oral side-effects of medications used to treat multiple sclerosis. Aust Dent J. 2017 Sep;62(3):331-336. doi: 10.1111/adj.12510. Epub 2017 May 31. PMID: 28276076.

increase viral load. Both THC and CBD are immune-suppressants [363] as well as Curcumin [364], Vitamin D [365], and GABA [366]. Gaba also regulates the release of pro-inflammatory cytokines [367].

Cannabinoids have the potential to slow down or prevent SARS-COV-2 replication in the lungs [368]. It has also been proposed that vitamin d [369], curcumin [370], and GABA [371] can also reduce lung injury. These studies have not been fully investigated.

Also, since blood sugar is a factor, it should be mentioned that all of these supplements have a positive impact on blood glucose. Cannabis [372], Vitamin D [373], Curcumin [374], and GABA [375]. Since blood sugar makes all of these biomarkers worse, and COVID-19 causes high blood sugar, even among those who don't have diabetes [376], this reduction in blood sugar by these supplements should, at least partially, reverse this effect.

According to the data in this ongoing study, these supplements also suppress substances related to viral load, organ damage, blood coagulation, mental degradation, and sepsis. Thus a combined treatment strategy could be a powerful solution to the prevention, and/or treatment of SARS-COV-2 in this pandemic.

363 Hegde VL, Nagarkatti M, Nagarkatti PS. Cannabinoid receptor activation leads to massive mobilization of myeloid-derived suppressor cells with potent immunosuppressive properties. Eur J Immunol. 2010 Dec;40(12):3358-71. doi: 10.1002/eji.201040667. PMID: 21110319; PMCID: PMC3076065.

364 Shirley, Shawna A et al. "Curcumin prevents human dendritic cell response to immune stimulants." Biochemical and biophysical research communications vol. 374,3 (2008): 431-6. doi:10.1016/j.bbrc.2008.07.051

365 Schwarz A, Navid F, Sparwasser T, Clausen BE, Schwarz T. 1,25-dihydroxyvitamin D exerts similar immunosuppressive effects as UVR but is dispensable for local UVR-induced immunosuppression. J Invest Dermatol. 2012 Dec;132(12):2762-9. doi: 10.1038/jid.2012.238. Epub 2012 Aug 2. PMID: 22854622.

366 Bhandage AK, Jin Z, Korol SV, Shen Q, Pei Y, Deng Q, Espes D, Carlsson PO, Kamali-Moghaddam M, Birnir B. GABA Regulates Release of Inflammatory Cytokines From Peripheral Blood Mononuclear Cells and CD4+ T Cells and Is Immunosuppressive in Type 1 Diabetes. EBioMedicine. 2018 Apr;30:283-294. doi: 10.1016/j.ebiom.2018.03.019. Epub 2018 Mar 28. PMID: 29627388; PMCID: PMC5952354.

367 Bhandage AK, Jin Z, Korol SV, Shen Q, Pei Y, Deng Q, Espes D, Carlsson PO, Kamali-Moghaddam M, Birnir B. GABA Regulates Release of Inflammatory Cytokines From Peripheral Blood Mononuclear Cells and CD4+ T Cells and Is Immunosuppressive in Type 1 Diabetes. EBioMedicine. 2018 Apr;30:283-294. doi: 10.1016/j.ebiom.2018.03.019. Epub 2018 Mar 28. PMID: 29627388; PMCID: PMC5952354.

368 Rosner M, et al. Cannabidiol Inhibits SARS-CoV-2 Replication and Promotes the Host Innate Immune Response. bioRxiv, 2021. doi: https://doi.org/10.1101/2021.03.10.432967

369 Xiao D, Li X, Su X, Mu D, Qu Y. Could SARS-CoV-2-induced lung injury be attenuated by vitamin D? Int J Infect Dis. 2021 Jan;102:196-202. doi: 10.1016/j.ijid.2020.10.059. Epub 2020 Oct 28. PMID: 33129966; PMCID: PMC7591873.

370 Zahedipour F, Hosseini SA, Sathyapalan T, Majeed M, Jamialahmadi T, Al-Rasadi K, Banach M, Sahebkar A. Potential effects of curcumin in the treatment of COVID-19 infection. Phytother Res. 2020 Nov;34(11):2911-2920. doi: 10.1002/ptr.6738. Epub 2020 Jun 23. PMID: 32430996; PMCID: PMC7276879.

371 Tian J, Middleton B, Kaufman DL. GABAA-Receptor Agonists Limit Pneumonitis and Death in Murine Coronavirus-Infected Mice. Viruses. 2021 May 23;13(6):966. doi: 10.3390/v13060966. PMID: 34071034; PMCID: PMC8224554.

372 Penner EA, Buettner H, Mittleman MA. The impact of marijuana use on glucose, insulin, and insulin resistance among US adults. Am J Med. 2013 Jul;126(7):583-9. doi: 10.1016/j.amjmed.2013.03.002. Epub 2013 May 15. PMID: 23684393.

373 Benetti E, Mastrocola R, Chiazza F, Nigro D, D'Antona G, Bordano V, et al. (2018) Effects of vitamin D on insulin resistance and myosteatosis in diet-induced obese mice. PLoS ONE 13(1): e0189707. https://doi.org/10.1371/journal.pone.0189707

374 Marton, Ledyane Taynara et al. "The Effects of Curcumin on Diabetes Mellitus: A Systematic Review." Frontiers in endocrinology vol. 12 669448. 3 May. 2021, doi:10.3389/fendo.2021.669448

375 Nakagawa T, Yokozawa T, Kim HJ, Shibahara N. Protective effects of gamma-aminobutyric acid in rats with streptozotocin-induced diabetes. J Nutr Sci Vitaminol (Tokyo). 2005 Aug;51(4):278-82. doi: 10.3177/jnsv.51.278. PMID: 16262002.

376 Carrasco-Sánchez FJ, López-Carmona MD, Martínez-Marcos FJ, Pérez-Belmonte LM, Hidalgo-Jiménez A, Buonaiuto V, Suárez Fernández C, Freire Castro SJ, Luordo D, Pesqueira Fontan PM, Blázquez Encinar JC, Magallanes Gamboa JO, de la Peña Fernández A, Torres Peña JD, Fernández Solà J, Napal Lecumberri JJ, Amorós Martínez F, Guisado Espartero ME, Jorge Ripper C, Gómez Méndez R, Vicente López N, Román Bernal B, Rojano Rivero MG, Ramos Rincón JM, Gómez Huelgas R; SEMI-COVID-19 Network. Admission hyperglycaemia as a predictor of mortality in patients hospitalized with COVID-19 regardless of diabetes status: data from the Spanish SEMI-COVID-19 Registry. Ann Med. 2021 Dec;53(1):103-116. doi: 10.1080/07853890.2020.1836566. PMID: 33063540; PMCID: PMC7651248.

Considerations

Clinical trials should begin on a combination of these supplements, while carbohydrates are reduced. If clinical trials replicate lab results, a combination of these herbs, vitamins, or supplements could be used as an emergency COVID-19 treatment. Also, as long these supplements are used responsibly, they could be taken as a preventive measure.

Hospital admissions of cannabis users for COVID-19 reveal lower inflammatory biomarkers [377], which adds to the evidence this treatment could work.

Some clinical trials on vitamin D do show a decline in biomarkers, such as cytokines, but not significantly [378]. Sugar intake and glucose levels may have skewed these results, or this is an argument for a combined treatment strategy using all of these supplements.

Cannabinol (CBD), Tetrahydrocannabinol (THC)

Because cannabinoids can affect the Cytochrome P450 enzyme [379] which prevents some medications from either being absorbed, or causes their effects to be enhanced, the advice of a physician should be sought, if CBD or THC is combined with any prescription medications.

Oral absorption of CBD is only about 6% bio-availability [380]. This may make vaping the best option for some people to fully absorb these drugs. The CDC has recommended against vaping during COVID, yet the National Institutes of Health (NIH) acknowledges CBD could be *a treatment for COVID-19.* It must be noted that any of these risks are primarily based on studies on vaping nicotine, or contaminates found in unregulated CBD or THC vape pens [381]. Suppressing cytokines, and other factors are important enough to far outweigh any risks vaping has on the lungs. Vaporization of butane-free CBD concentrate may be the safest, and best delivery method. A device that gently heats this concentrate is available.

Studies since the 1970's have demonstrated that even inhaling cannabis smoke has a positive effect on asthma [382], and could be a treatment for COPD [383]. Cannabis is a bronchodilator [384], unlike nicotine, which is a bronchoconstrictor [385]. Any negative effects should be of far less concern than the potential of cytokine suppression, which causes the COVID-19 pneumonia, and lung damage.

---

377 Shover CM, Yan P, Jackson NJ, Buhr RG, Fulcher JA, Tashkin DP, Barjaktarevic I. Cannabis consumption is associated with lower COVID-19 severity among hospitalized patients: a retrospective cohort analysis. J Cannabis Res. 2022 Aug 5;4(1):46. doi: 10.1186/s42238-022-00152-x. PMID: 35932069; PMCID: PMC9356466.

378 Yusupov E, Li-Ng M, Pollack S, Yeh JK, Mikhail M, Aloia JF. Vitamin d and serum cytokines in a randomized clinical trial. Int J Endocrinol. 2010;2010:305054. doi: 10.1155/2010/305054. Epub 2010 Aug 12. PMID: 20871847; PMCID: PMC2943086.

379 Zendulka O, Dovrtělová G, Nosková K, Turjap M, Šulcová A, Hanuš L, Juřica J. Cannabinoids and Cytochrome P450 Interactions. Curr Drug Metab. 2016;17(3):206-26. doi: 10.2174/1389200217666151210142051. PMID: 26651971.

380 Perucca E, Bialer M. Critical Aspects Affecting Cannabidiol Oral Bioavailability and Metabolic Elimination, and Related Clinical Implications. CNS Drugs. 2020 Aug;34(8):795-800. doi: 10.1007/s40263-020-00741-5. PMID: 32504461.

381 Meehan-Atrash J, Rahman I. Cannabis Vaping: Existing and Emerging Modalities, Chemistry, and Pulmonary Toxicology. Chem Res Toxicol. 2021 Oct 18;34(10):2169-2179. doi: 10.1021/acs.chemrestox.1c00290. Epub 2021 Oct 8. PMID: 34622654; PMCID: PMC8882064.

382 Hartley JP, Nogrady SG, Seaton A. Bronchodilator effect of delta1-tetrahydrocannabinol. Br J Clin Pharmacol. 1978 Jun;5(6):523-5. doi: 10.1111/j.1365-2125.1978.tb01667.x. PMID: 656294; PMCID: PMC1429361.

383 Abdallah SJ, Smith BM, Ware MA, Moore M, Li PZ, Bourbeau J, Jensen D. Effect of Vaporized Cannabis on Exertional Breathlessness and Exercise Endurance in Advanced Chronic Obstructive Pulmonary Disease. A Randomized Controlled Trial. Ann Am Thorac Soc. 2018 Oct;15(10):1146-1158. doi: 10.1513/AnnalsATS.201803-198OC. PMID: 30049223.

384 Hartley JP, Nogrady SG, Seaton A. Bronchodilator effect of delta1-tetrahydrocannabinol. Br J Clin Pharmacol. 1978 Jun;5(6):523-5. doi: 10.1111/j.1365-2125.1978.tb01667.x. PMID: 656294; PMCID: PMC1429361.

385 Lee LY, Lin RL, Khosravi M, Xu F. Reflex bronchoconstriction evoked by inhaled nicotine aerosol in guinea pigs: role of the nicotinic acetylcholine receptor. J Appl Physiol (1985). 2018 Jul 1;125(1):117-123. doi: 10.1152/japplphysiol.01039.2017. Epub 2018 Jan 25. PMID: 29369741; PMCID: PMC6086971.

As cited in this document, cannabinoids also have been shown to reduce substances related to blood coagulation, which constricts oxygen supply, and breathing in severe COVID.

There have been some studies that have linked THC to schizophrenic episodes, but a review of all studies found no evidence [386]. Nevertheless, first use cannabis does raise dopamine levels, but continued use blunts dopamine response [387]. For this reason, either first use or sporadic use could trigger a first-event schizophrenic episode—at any dosage. However, this is also true of many prescription drugs, over the counter drugs, and herbal supplements [388].

Although THC raises CCL11 [389], and CCL11 has also found to be raised in schizophrenics [390], this is due to a Th1/Th2 imbalance that raises cytokine levels. IP-10/CXCL10 have also been found to be raised in all people with schizophrenia, and bi-polar disorder [391]. Increased levels of TARC/CCL17 were also found in schizophrenics [392].

CBD lowers CCL11 [393], and both THC and CBD lower TARC/CCL17 [394]. Since THC lowers IP-10/CXCL10 [395], this explains why higher CCL11 levels have not led to noticeable increase in schizophrenia diagnosis in states that have legalized Cannabis.

Some argue that increased hospitalizations for cannabis related events in states such as Colorado indicate cannabis is a schizophrenic trigger [396], but these episodes of paranoia can be understood as transient, possibly due to the overdose of edibles, or reactions among first time users.

There were also lower levels of CCL24, or eotaxin-2 [397] among schizophrenics. The Cannabinoid receptor CB-2 controls CCL24 [398]. This is the receptor most influenced by CBD. All of these facts reveal this is a complicated issue, not as simple as an elevation in one chemokine.

386 Ahmed S, Roth RM, Stanciu CN, Brunette MF. The Impact of THC and CBD in Schizophrenia: A Systematic Review. Front Psychiatry. 2021 Jul 23;12:694394. doi: 10.3389/fpsyt.2021.694394. PMID: 34366924; PMCID: PMC8343183.

387 Bloomfield MA, Ashok AH, Volkow ND, Howes OD. The effects of Δ9-tetrahydrocannabinol on the dopamine system. Nature. 2016 Nov 17;539(7629):369-377. doi: 10.1038/nature20153. PMID: 27853201; PMCID: PMC5123717.

388 Sexton JD, Pronchik DJ. Diphenhydramine-induced psychosis with therapeutic doses. Am J Emerg Med. 1997 Sep;15(5):548-9. doi: 10.1016/s0735-6757(97)90212-6. PMID: 9270406.

389 Fernandez-Egea E, Scoriels L, Theegala S, Giro M, Ozanne SE, Burling K, Jones PB. Cannabis use is associated with increased CCL11 plasma levels in young healthy volunteers. Prog Neuropsychopharmacol Biol Psychiatry. 2013 Oct 1;46:25-8. doi: 10.1016/j.pnpbp.2013.06.011. Epub 2013 Jun 29. PMID: 23820464.

390 Teixeira AL, Reis HJ, Nicolato R, Brito-Melo G, Correa H, Teixeira MM, Romano-Silva MA. Increased serum levels of CCL11/eotaxin in schizophrenia. Prog Neuropsychopharmacol Biol Psychiatry. 2008 Apr 1;32(3):710-4. doi: 10.1016/j.pnpbp.2007.11.019. Epub 2007 Nov 23. PMID: 18096286.

391 Teixeira AL, Gama CS, Rocha NP, Teixeira MM. Revisiting the Role of Eotaxin-1/CCL11 in Psychiatric Disorders. Front Psychiatry. 2018 Jun 14;9:241. doi: 10.3389/fpsyt.2018.00241. PMID: 29962972; PMCID: PMC6010544.

392 Malmqvist A, Schwieler L, Orhan F, Fatouros-Bergman H, Bauer M, Flyckt L, Cervenka S, Engberg G, Piehl F; Karolinska Schizophrenia Project (KaSP) consortium, Erhardt S. Increased peripheral levels of TARC/CCL17 in first episode psychosis patients. Schizophr Res. 2019 Aug;210:221-227. doi: 10.1016/j.schres.2018.12.033. Epub 2019 Jan 3. PMID: 30612841.

393 Rachayon M, Jirakran K, Sodsai P, Klinchanhom S, Sughondhabirom A, Plaimas K, Suratanee A, Maes M. In Vitro Effects of Cannabidiol on Activated Immune-Inflammatory Pathways in Major Depressive Patients and Healthy Controls. Pharmaceuticals (Basel). 2022 Mar 26;15(4):405. doi: 10.3390/ph15040405. PMID: 35455402; PMCID: PMC9032852.

394 Massimini M, Dalle Vedove E, Bachetti B, Di Pierro F, Ribecco C, D'Addario C, Pucci M. Polyphenols and Cannabidiol Modulate Transcriptional Regulation of Th1/Th2 Inflammatory Genes Related to Canine Atopic Dermatitis. Front Vet Sci. 2021 Mar 5;8:606197. doi: 10.3389/fvets.2021.606197. PMID: 33763461; PMCID: PMC7982812.

395 Henriquez JE, Bach AP, Matos-Fernandez KM, Crawford RB, Kaminski NE. Δ9-Tetrahydrocannabinol (THC) Impairs CD8+ T Cell-Mediated Activation of Astrocytes. J Neuroimmune Pharmacol. 2020 Dec;15(4):863-874. doi: 10.1007/s11481-020-09912-z. Epub 2020 Mar 26. PMID: 32215844; PMCID: PMC7529688.

396 Crocker CE, Carter AJE, Emsley JG, Magee K, Atkinson P, Tibbo PG. When Cannabis Use Goes Wrong: Mental Health Side Effects of Cannabis Use That Present to Emergency Services. Front Psychiatry. 2021 Feb 15;12:640222. doi: 10.3389/fpsyt.2021.640222. PMID: 33658953; PMCID: PMC7917124.

397 Teixeira AL, Gama CS, Rocha NP, Teixeira MM. Revisiting the Role of Eotaxin-1/CCL11 in Psychiatric Disorders. Front Psychiatry. 2018 Jun 14;9:241. doi: 10.3389/fpsyt.2018.00241. PMID: 29962972; PMCID: PMC6010544.

398 Palazuelos J, Davoust N, Julien B, Hatterer E, Aguado T, Mechoulam R, Benito C, Romero J, Silva A, Guzmán M, Nataf S, Galve-Roperh I. The CB(2) cannabinoid receptor controls myeloid progenitor trafficking: involvement in the pathogenesis of an animal model of multiple sclerosis. J Biol Chem. 2008 May 9;283(19):13320-9. doi: 10.1074/jbc.M707960200. Epub 2008 Mar 11. PMID: 18334483.

CBD in high doses has raised an enzyme in horses [399] that causes liver damage, also raised in COVID-19 [400]. Although there is no evidence CBD causes this elevation in humans, this could be possible at extremely high doses.

There also may be a risk upon sudden discontinuation of Cannabis. Cannabis is a blood thinner, as Warfarin. Sudden discontinuation of Warfarin can cause a stroke [401] and it can increase stroke risk with certain conditions [402].There have been reports of rare heart attacks [403], strokes [404], and even death [405] upon sudden discontinuation of regular, high dose cannabis, or a rare reaction due to a medical condition. However, it should be noted that some prescription drugs, or herbal supplements can also trigger these rare events [406].

Warfarin is used for COVID-19, despite these slight risks. For the same reason, there should be no apprehension using cannabinoids as a treatment. Furthermore, anyone who uses cannabis on a regular basis—especially high potency cannabis—should *never* discontinue suddenly (which happens during hospitalization.) This risks a "rebound effect," with the potential to cause blood clots. However, hospitalized cannabis patients (who would discontinue) had similar outcomes, but had lower inflammation when admitted [407].

Curcumin

The proper dose of curcumin has protected against liver injury in lab animals[408]. However, extremely high doses has caused rare cases of liver injury [409].

It is possible curcumin can interact with prescription medications [410].

399 Watkins PB, Church RJ, Li J, Knappertz V. Cannabidiol and Abnormal Liver Chemistries in Healthy Adults: Results of a Phase I Clinical Trial. Clin Pharmacol Ther. 2021 May;109(5):1224-1231. doi: 10.1002/cpt.2071. Epub 2020 Nov 21. PMID: 33022751; PMCID: PMC8246741.

400 Kasapoglu B, Yozgat A, Tanoglu A, Can G, Sakin YS, Kekilli M. Gamma-glutamyl-transferase may predict COVID-19 outcomes in hospitalised patients. Int J Clin Pract. 2021 Dec;75(12):e14933. doi: 10.1111/ijcp.14933. Epub 2021 Oct 8. PMID: 34605109; PMCID: PMC8646326.

401 Spivey CA, Liu X, Qiao Y, Mardekian J, Parker RB, Phatak H, Masseria C, Kachroo S, Abdulsattar Y, Wang J. Stroke associated with discontinuation of warfarin therapy for atrial fibrillation. Curr Med Res Opin. 2015 Nov;31(11):2021-9. doi: 10.1185/03007995.2015.1082995. Epub 2015 Sep 21. PMID: 26390258.

402 https://www.medicinenet.com/script/main/art.asp?articlekey=175827

403 Richards JR, Blohm E, Toles KA, Jarman AF, Ely DF, Elder JW. The association of cannabis use and cardiac dysrhythmias: a systematic review. Clin Toxicol (Phila). 2020 Sep;58(9):861-869. doi: 10.1080/15563650.2020.1743847. Epub 2020 Apr 8. PMID: 32267189.

404 Trojak B, Leclerq S, Meille V, Khoumri C, Chauvet-Gelinier JC, Giroud M, Bonin B, Gisselmann A. Stroke with neuropsychiatric sequelae after cannabis use in a man: a case report. J Med Case Rep. 2011 Jun 30;5:264. doi: 10.1186/1752-1947-5-264. PMID: 21718541; PMCID: PMC3148997.

405 Drummer OH, Gerostamoulos D, Woodford NW. Cannabis as a cause of death: A review. Forensic Sci Int. 2019 May;298:298-306. doi: 10.1016/j.forsciint.2019.03.007. Epub 2019 Mar 14. PMID: 30925348.

406 Page RL 2nd, O'Bryant CL, Cheng D, Dow TJ, Ky B, Stein CM, Spencer AP, Trupp RJ, Lindenfeld J; American Heart Association Clinical Pharmacology and Heart Failure and Transplantation Committees of the Council on Clinical Cardiology; Council on Cardiovascular Surgery and Anesthesia; Council on Cardiovascular and Stroke Nursing; and Council on Quality of Care and Outcomes Research. Drugs That May Cause or Exacerbate Heart Failure: A Scientific Statement From the American Heart Association. Circulation. 2016 Aug 9;134(6):e32-69. doi: 10.1161/CIR.0000000000000426. Epub 2016 Jul 11. Erratum in: Circulation. 2016 Sep 20;134(12):e261. PMID: 27400984.

407 Shover CM, Yan P, Jackson NJ, Buhr RG, Fulcher JA, Tashkin DP, Barjaktarevic I. Cannabis consumption is associated with lower COVID-19 severity among hospitalized patients: a retrospective cohort analysis. J Cannabis Res. 2022 Aug 5;4(1):46. doi: 10.1186/s42238-022-00152-x. PMID: 35932069; PMCID: PMC9356466.

408 Fu Y, Zheng S, Lin J, Ryerse J, Chen A. Curcumin protects the rat liver from CCl4-caused injury and fibrogenesis by attenuating oxidative stress and suppressing inflammation. Mol Pharmacol. 2008 Feb;73(2):399-409. doi: 10.1124/mol.107.039818. Epub 2007 Nov 15. PMID: 18006644.

409 Somanawat K, Thong-Ngam D, Klaikeaw N. Curcumin attenuated paracetamol overdose induced hepatitis. World J Gastroenterol. 2013 Mar 28;19(12):1962-7. doi: 10.3748/wjg.v19.i12.1962. PMID: 23569342; PMCID: PMC3613112.

410 Bahramsoltani R, Rahimi R, Farzaei MH. Pharmacokinetic interactions of curcuminoids with conventional drugs: A review. J Ethnopharmacol. 2017 Sep 14;209:1-12. doi: 10.1016/j.jep.2017.07.022. Epub 2017 Jul 19. PMID: 28734960.

Vitamin D
There have been a few reports of an interactions between vitamin D and GABA, but this data is limited. Vitamin D, which is an anticoagulant, can cause blood coagulation at high doses possibly by a decrease in Thrombospodin-1 [411], which is also decreased in COVID-19 [412].

Gaba

Gaba has caused drug interactions [413] and has potential side effects. It can possibly trigger and/or aggravate schizophrenia [414]. However, as stated, so can many prescription drugs, and over the counter medications, if someone has this genetic condition.

These facts do not make these supplements any more dangerous than prescription drugs, if taken in recommended doses. Since these supplements can be taken together, the *lowest* effective dose of each should be the goal of clinical studies, combined with a reduction in sugars and carbs. This should reduce potential reactions or side effects at extremely high doses. Of course, without clinical trials covering a broad spectrum of candidates, the potential of this treatment will never be known.

Russell Redden
8/01/22

For a complete list of substances being reviewed in this ongoing study: **COVID19SciencePortal.com**

411 Amarasekera AT, Assadi-Khansari B, Liu S, Black M, Dymmott G, Rogers NM, Sverdlov AL, Horowitz JD, Ngo DTM. Vitamin D supplementation lowers thrombospondin-1 levels and blood pressure in healthy adults. PLoS One. 2017 May 10;12(5):e0174435. doi: 10.1371/journal.pone.0174435. PMID: 28489857; PMCID: PMC5425007.
412 Ward SE, Fogarty H, Karampini E, Lavin M, Schneppenheim S, Dittmer R, Morrin H, Glavey S, Ni Cheallaigh C, Bergin C, Martin-Loeches I, Mallon PW, Curley GF, Baker RI, Budde U, O'Sullivan JM, O'Donnell JS; Irish COVID-19 Vasculopathy Study (iCVS) investigators. ADAMTS13 regulation of VWF multimer distribution in severe COVID-19. J Thromb Haemost. 2021 Aug;19(8):1914-1921. doi: 10.1111/jth.15409. Epub 2021 Jun 20. PMID: 34053187; PMCID: PMC8237059.
413 Olsen RW. GABA-drug interactions. Prog Drug Res. 1987;31:223-41. doi: 10.1007/978-3-0348-9289-6_6. PMID: 2449703.
414 Meldrum B. Pharmacology of GABA. Clin Neuropharmacol. 1982;5(3):293-316. doi: 10.1097/00002826-198205030-00004. PMID: 6214305.